The Gut Health Plan
© 2024 Future Publishing Limited

Future Books is an imprint of Future PLC
Quay House, The Ambury, Bath, BA1 1UA

A catalogue record for this book is
available from the British Library.

ISBN 978-1-80521-765-7 hardback

The paper holds full FSC certification
and accreditation.

Printed in China by C&C Offset Printing Co. Ltd.
for Future PLC

**Interested in Foreign Rights to publish this title?
Email us at:**
licensing@futurenet.com

Editor
Philippa Grafton

Art Editor
Lora Barnes

Contributors
**Edoardo Albert, Jamie Frier, Zara Gaspar,
Eva Gizowska, Lucy Gornall, Ailsa Harvey,
Ali Horsfall, Kate Marsh, Faye M Smith,
Louise Pyne, Eleanor Vousden, Debra Waters**

Senior Art Editor
Stephen Williams

Head of Art & Design
Greg Whitaker

Editorial Director
Jon White

Managing Director
Grainne McKenna

Production Project Manager
Matthew Eglinton

Global Business Development Manager
Jennifer Smith

Head of Future International & Bookazines
Tim Mathers

Cover images
Getty Images

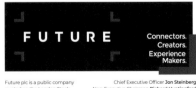

Future plc is a public company
quoted on the London Stock
Exchange
(symbol: FUTR)
www.futureplc.com

Chief Executive Officer **Jon Steinberg**
Non-Executive Chairman **Richard Huntingford**
Chief Financial and Strategy Officer **Penny Ladkin-Brand**

Tel +44 (0)1225 442 244

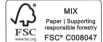

The

GUT HEALTH

Plan

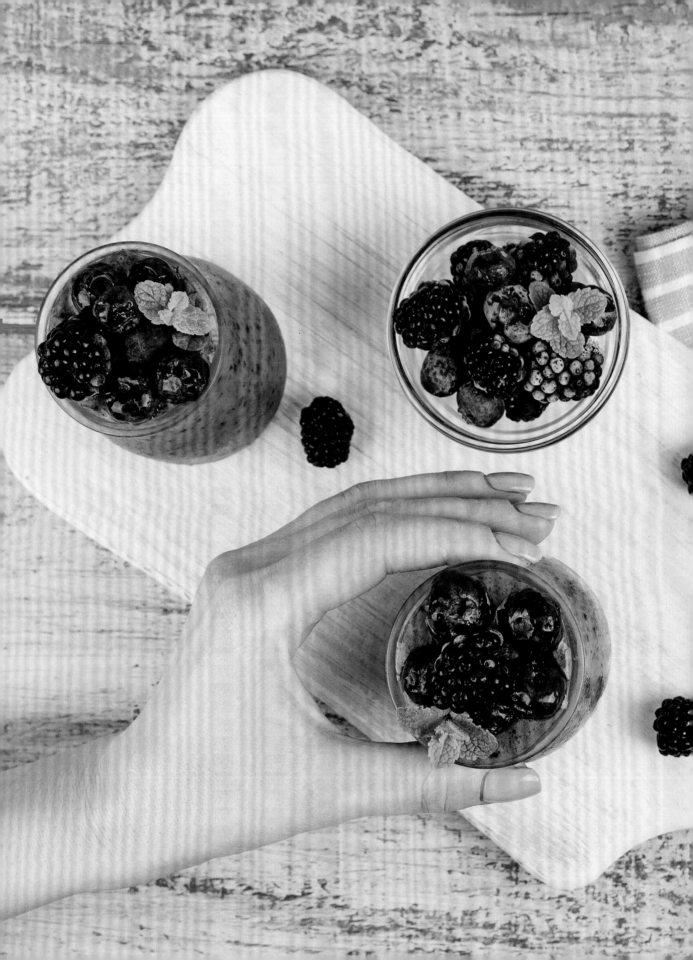

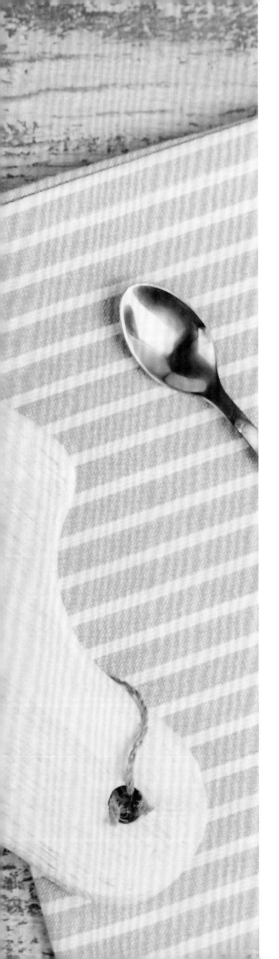

Welcome

The health of our insides impacts more than just how bloated we feel; research shows that a healthy gut can improve our immune system, physical appearance and even our mental wellbeing. But everybody's gut is different and what might work for one person won't necessarily work for another. In this brand-new title, The Gut Health Plan, find out how to understand your own microbiome, from what dishes don't agree with you to the foods that your gut has been crying out for. With dozens of gut-friendly recipes, this is the essential guide to improving your health from the inside out!

Contents

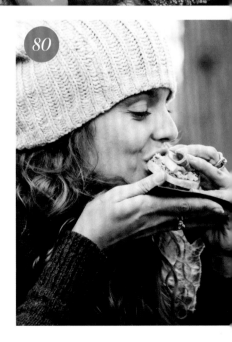

Science

58

Diet

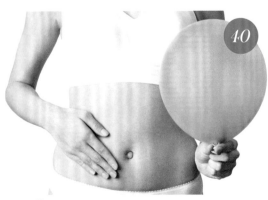

40

80

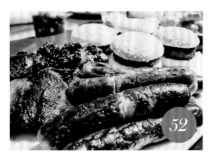

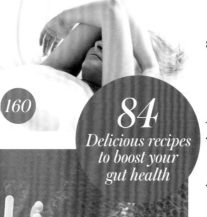

52

160

Lifestyle

16

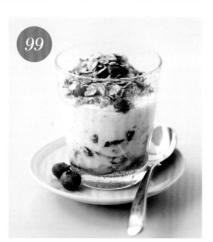

99

12

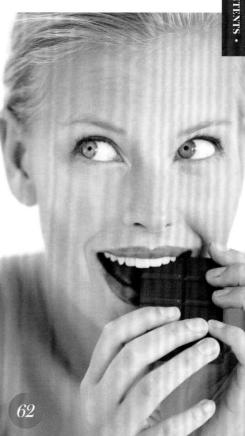

62

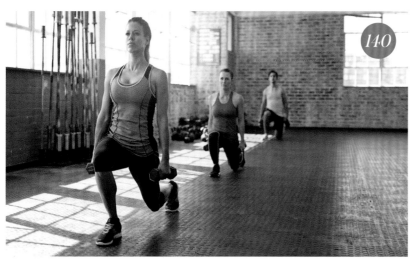

140

Science

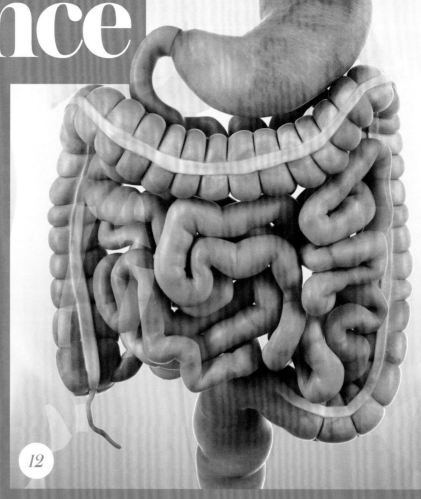

12

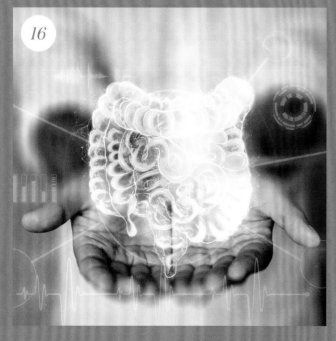

16

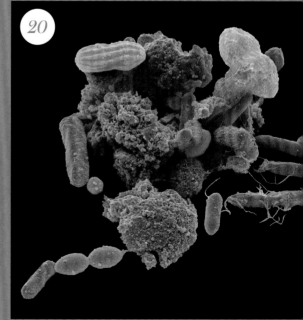

20

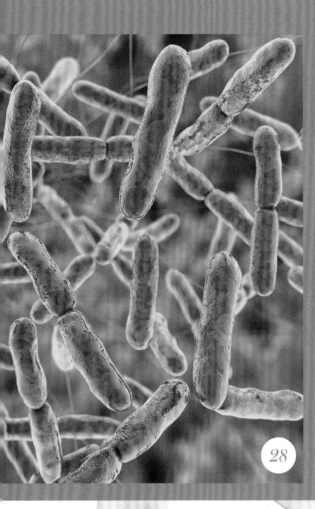

28

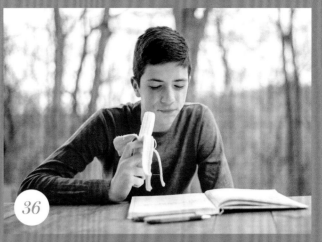

36

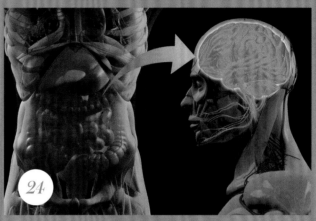

24

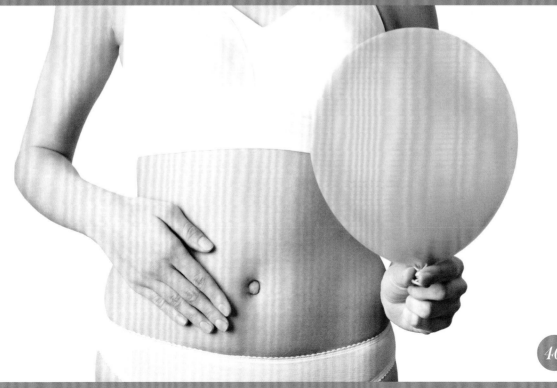

40

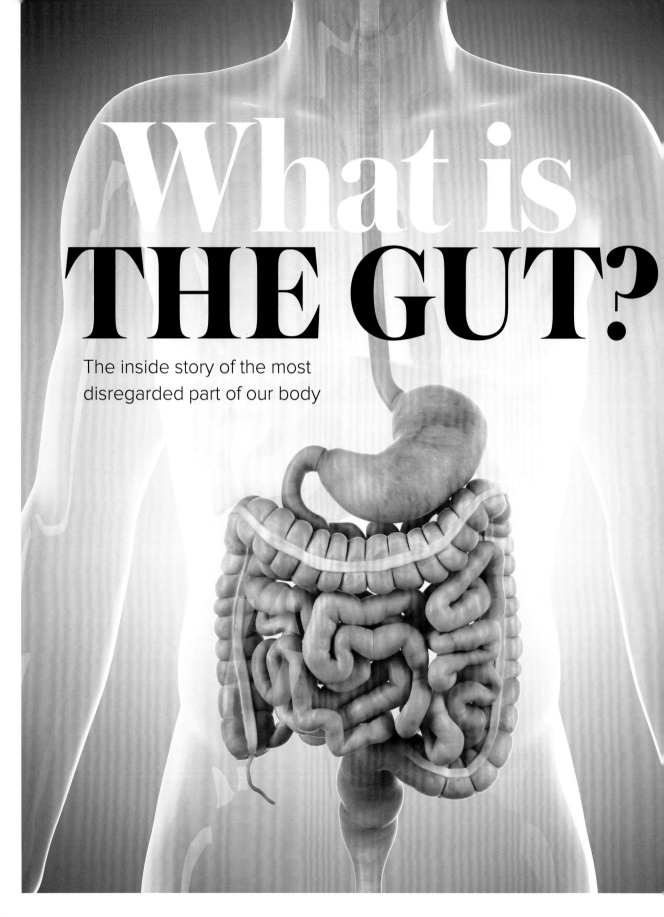

What is THE GUT?

The inside story of the most disregarded part of our body

What is the gut? The most straightforward answer is that it is the tube that runs from your mouth to your bottom. The gut takes the lovely, tasty food you chew and swallow, pushes it through the body and expels it out the other end. By which time it's no longer quite so appetising.

It's an unglamorous job compared to our other important systems. We know the gut is fundamental because it's there almost from the beginning of life, when the fertilised egg starts to develop in the mother's womb. One of the first things the fertilised cell does as it grows and divides is to split into what are basically three tubes. The first has a little bulge in the middle, which a little later starts to beat: yes, it's our heart. The rest of the tube develops into the whole cardiovascular system: lungs, blood vessels, our bodily engine. The second tube also starts off with a bulge in the middle, but it moves up to the top, becoming our brain, while the rest of the tube develops into the nervous system, our body's command and control system.

The third tube becomes the gut. It's as basic to our functioning as our hearts and our brains, although when faced with the choice of whether we would lose our heart, brain or appendix, the answer seems to be a no-brainer. So what makes the gut so important?

THE GATE

The gut begins in your mouth. Since we stare into it every time we brush our teeth, it might seem the best-known part of the gut, but it has many secrets and not a few surprises. Its first four surprises are the little bumps, two on the walls of the mouth and two under the tongue, flanking the lingual frenulum, the strip of

'Saliva also contains a potent painkiller, opiorphin, which is stronger than morphine'

tissue tying your tongue to the floor of the mouth. These are called the parotid papillae, and they are the taps through which the salivary glands pipe up to one litre of saliva into the mouth each day.

The salivary glands filter red blood corpuscles from the blood but send much of the rest of the liquid through into our mouths, which means that saliva can be used to test for lots of stuff from our immune system.

Saliva also contains a potent painkiller, opiorphin, which is stronger than morphine, that was only discovered in 2006. Of course, in the normal course of events our saliva only contains tiny amounts of opiorphin or we'd all be permanently high, but even in tiny amounts it helps counteract the extreme pain sensitivity of the mouth, which ranks alongside our fingers in nerve density. Saliva also has antibacterial properties, which is why animals lick their wounds.

THE WAY DOWN

The oesophagus – the tube down from the mouth to the stomach – has one of the most difficult jobs in the body. Design constraints mean that it has a

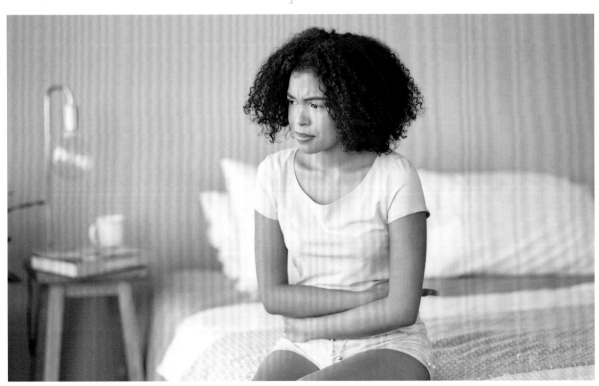

double function in its upper reaches, conveying air to our lungs and food to our stomachs. Sending air to the lungs produces burps and flatulence. Sending food to the lungs can kill. Swallowing is an intricate dance, where the bolus, the lump of masticated food, is pushed to the back of the mouth. Then the nasal cavity is closed off by the soft palate rising, the larynx moves up and forward, the epiglottis shuts off the airway to the lungs (stopping you breathing), the pharynx sends the bolus down the throat and the upper oesophageal sphincter muscle opens, allowing the bolus through, and then closes again.

Wavelike contractions of the oesophagus move the bolus down to the stomach and when it reaches the stomach, the lower oesophageal sphincter opens to let the bolus in and then closes again.

STOMACH TROUBLE

If you have a stomach ache and, when asked where the pain is, point somewhere in the region of your navel, then the pain isn't in the stomach. In fact, the stomach sits quite high in the body, beginning below the left nipple and ending under the right ribcage. The stomach is a lopsided organ, shaped rather like a kidney bean, with the oesophagus feeding into the side of the stomach, albeit near the top; there's a little bulge of stomach above the point where the oesophagus joins on.

The position of the stomach entrance is deliberate: it reduces the pressure on the oesophagus from the stomach contents when our abdomen presses against it while also allowing liquids to drop straight down the short side of the stomach into the small intestine. Solid foods are directed towards the stomach's holding area for further work before going on.

In fact, the two sides of the stomach are specialised, with the long outer curve dealing with food and the short inner curve dealing with liquids. As the top of the stomach lies above the point where the oesophagus enters it, gas can rise and get trapped in the top portion of

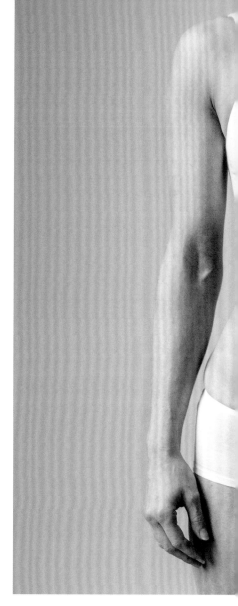

> 'The internal surface area of the small intestine is about 30 square metres'

the stomach. If troubled by trapped wind at night, an easy way to help is to roll over on to your left-hand side, so that the trapped air can go up and out.

THE SMALL INTESTINE

It's not so small. The small intestine winds for between three and six convoluted metres in our middles, curling backward and forwards. The inside of the small intestine, the part in contact with our food, is covered in folds and little digits that stick their fingers into the passing chyme, the semi-digested food going past them. There are so many of these villi and folds that the internal surface area of the small intestine is about 30 square metres – like the Tardis, we are bigger on the inside than the outside.

The small intestine has three parts: the short duodenum at its start; the jejunum, the mid-section of the small intestine, which is about 2.5 metres in length; and the ileum, approximately three metres long, which joins on to the large intestine. The duodenum produces enzymes that breakdown much of the chyme into easily absorbable molecules.

As the chyme enters the duodenum, the duodenal papilla, which is like the salivary papillae of the mouth, squirts it with digestive juices: enzymes and fat solvents. The chyme then passes into the jejunum, where the sugars, amino acids and fatty acids that have been produced by our digestive juices are absorbed into the bloodstream. What hasn't already been absorbed passes into the ileum, which is responsible for taking up bile acids and left behind nutrients. What's left over goes into the large intestine.

THE LARGE INTESTINE

The small intestine's bigger brother does not wind and wiggle like its junior. Instead, it starts low, goes up the right side of our body, crosses the abdomen and then goes down the left side before turning back towards the middle and aiming for the bottom. When looking at the body from the front, it appears to frame the small intestine. And indeed, that's what it does: it takes care of the business left over from the small intestine. The body is thorough in absorbing everything possible from the food it eats.

The small intestine does an excellent job of breaking down and absorbing the main parts of our diet, and it does this quickly too: a meal passes through our

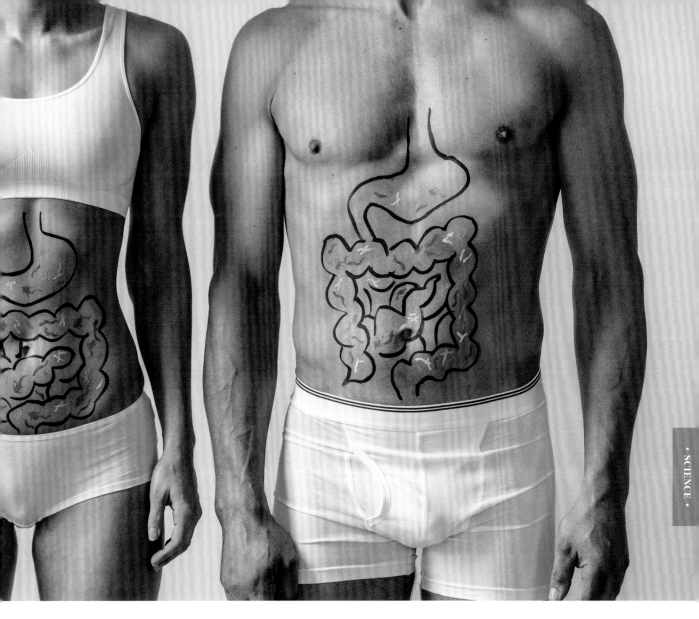

small intestine in four to eight hours. The large intestine takes longer: it ruminates on the leftovers for some 16 hours, sifting through whatever is left, including important minerals such as calcium, and vitamins B1 (thiamine), B2 (riboflavin) and B12.

To absorb these and other difficult-to-access substances, the large intestine works in concert with a huge and varied garden of gut bacteria. Our insides are a partnership between us and literally billions of bacteria, with most of these finding their home in the large intestine. The final metre of the large intestine absorbs water and salt, adjusting the amounts so that ideally, when what is left in the large intestine reaches the end

of the road, it can be pushed out with ease.

ARE YOU SITTING COMFORTABLY?

At the end of the tunnel, there are two sphincter muscles. One we can clamp shut if what's knocking is doing so at a completely inappropriate time. It's under our conscious control.

But the other one, the inner sphincter muscle, works as part of the gut and when the final leftovers – our faeces – reach it, the inner sphincter muscle opens to let a sample of what wants to come through into the small passage in between the two sphincter muscles. There, nerve cells inform our conscious

minds of what wants to come out: solid, gas or, sometimes, liquid. That's when we have to decide whether we can act upon the urge now, or if it has to be postponed to later.

Opening the outer sphincter muscle is a signal to the inner one that it's all right to let what's knocking through. But if we're talking to the Queen, we're more likely to squeeze that outer sphincter tightly. Doing so passes the message to the inner sphincter muscle: not now! So long as the internal situation is not desperate, it will accept the message, tighten up and wait until later. But in the end, what's left of what came in must come out. That so little does so is a testament to the efficiency of our gut.

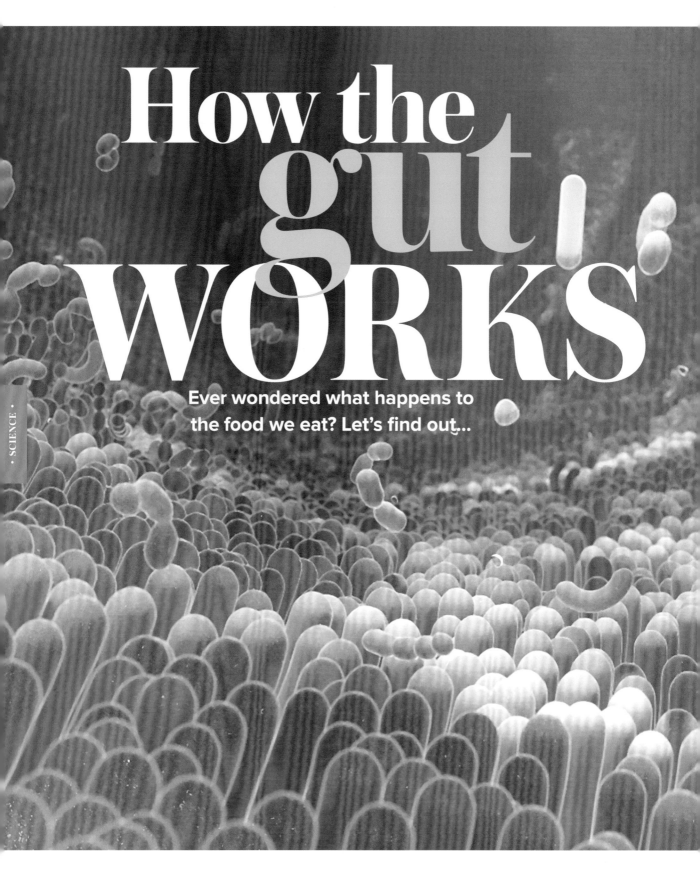

How the gut WORKS

Ever wondered what happens to the food we eat? Let's find out...

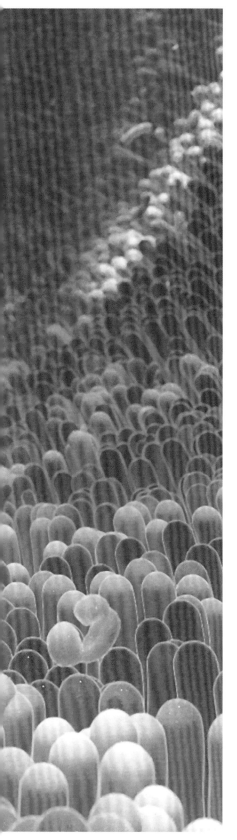

Humans are omnivores. Unlike cats, who can only survive by eating meat, or cows, who thrive on plants, we can eat everything: flesh, fowl, fruit, vegetable, and ideally a few minerals, too. It is the gut's job to take this incredible variety of foodstuffs and render it into fuel and the raw material for replacement parts.

An oil refinery takes just one source material, crude oil, and refines it into different grades of petrol and diesel. Our gut takes everything we drop into it (well, almost everything: there are a few times it will object to what we are trying to feed it and remove the offending contents in one almighty, convulsive heave) and converts it into a much wider variety of outputs. But how does it do this?

DIFFERENT TYPES OF MUSCLE

Our bodies are home to three different types of muscle. Lift a weight, sit down, scratch your nose: in all these cases it's skeletal (striated) muscle that's doing the work. It's called striated because, under a microscope, it looks like strips of muscle tissue. This type of muscle is under our conscious control.

Next, put your hand on your chest. The thumping you can feel is coming from your cardiac muscle. Like skeletal muscle, it looks striated under a microscope, but it's not under our conscious control — no one can stop their heart by willing it to stop.

Finally, there is smooth muscle, so called because it looks smooth under the microscope, and this makes up the walls of our gut. Rather than being under the control of the central nervous system, the

'To ensure we don't choke, the larynx and the epiglottis work in tandem'

gut is controlled by the enteric nervous system. This works so independently that even if the connection between the enteric nervous system and the brain is cut, it just keeps working.

This is not to say that our bodily and emotional states don't affect our gut; they clearly do, particularly when we are under great stress. But most of the time, the enteric nervous system quietly gets on with its job of regulating our gastrointestinal system, making sure that we have all that we need to carry on doing what we need to be doing.

EATING AND CHEWING

The first acts in the whole digestive circus take place in the mouth. There, two of the most extraordinary muscles in our bodies work together in a delicate dance to get food ready for delivery below. Our jaw muscle is the most powerful muscle in the body and, contrary to the common notion that the human bite is relatively puny, pound for pound we bite harder than our simian cousins, exerting a force between 1,100 and 1,300 Newtons when using our molars. Our chewing power, using the molars, is considerably greater than our biting strength, using the incisors and canines, but it still leaves us not that far behind the biting force of dogs. Given how hard we bite, it's no surprise that the tongue is the most flexible muscle in the body: it has to stay clear of those teeth when they chomp. We all know how painful it is when we get it wrong and accidentally bite our tongue.

Working together, jaws, teeth (tooth enamel is suitably the hardest substance in the body) and tongue turn the food into something that can be swallowed. The tongue comes into its own at this point, separating out about 20 millilitres of chewed food, which it impresses on the palate, triggering the swallow reflex.

GOING DOWN

Swallowing is a complex process. To ensure we don't choke, the larynx and the epiglottis work in tandem, the larynx moving up and forward while the epiglottis seals off the airway to the lungs to prevent food going the wrong way. The upper tract of our throat, up to the hollow at the base of the throat, is surrounded by striated muscle so we can feel food going down that far but beyond that, the bolus of masticated food enters the territory of the smooth muscle of the gut.

Waves of swelling, called propulsive peristalsis, push the bolus down the oesophagus to the stomach. The onwards motion is so powerful that even if we stood on our head and swallowed, the food would still get to the stomach. There's another sphincter muscle at the bottom of the oesophagus that seals off the stomach. When this gateway sphincter muscle feels the propulsive peristalsis above it in the oesophagus, it relaxes, opening for eight seconds to allow the bolus into the stomach before closing again. It takes five to ten seconds for food to make it from the back of the mouth to the stomach. The journey involves over 20 pairs of muscles, working in concert. And it's just the start of the journey.

THE TUMMY TUCKS IN

The stomach, alerted by the motion of the oesophagus and the opening of the

sphincter muscle, relaxes in preparation for the incoming load. Surrounded by smooth muscle, it can expand to hold remarkable amounts of food: a kilogram would be no problem for it. With the food safely contained, the stomach muscles proceed to give it a good kicking, bouncing it off the stomach walls in a process called retropulsion.

The stomach mixes the food, rather like a cement mixer, breaking it all down so that it's almost all reduced to tiny bits less than two millimetres across. How long food spends in the stomach depends on what it was. Simple carbohydrates and sugars can be moved on to the small intestine in an hour or less; more complex proteins, like a steak, might take four or five hours to be broken down properly.

THE LONG AND WINDING ROAD

When the stomach starts jumping – going into retropulsion – it warns the small intestine that more food will be coming through soon. The small intestine responds by shifting what's inside it along, making room for more.

With its vast internal surface area, the small intestine is where the great majority of the nutrients from our food are absorbed. The tiny villi are themselves covered with even tinier projections, the microvilli, through which most of the absorption of the sugars and amino acids takes place. The whole small intestine, and all its villi and microvilli, work in concert to keep the food, now a semi-fluid called chyme, moving along.

Having eaten, and digested, about an hour after the food has passed by, the small intestine begins to clean house, technically known as the migrating motor complex. This is what's responsible for the rumbling tummy sound if you're feeling hungry. The migrating motor complex moves bacteria out of the small intestine, where there should be few bacteria, to the rich bacterial pastures of the large intestine, while also stopping bacteria coming back in the opposite direction.

As such, the migrating motor complex plays an important role in the overall health of the small intestine. However, as soon as we eat something, the migrating motor complex stops, so constant

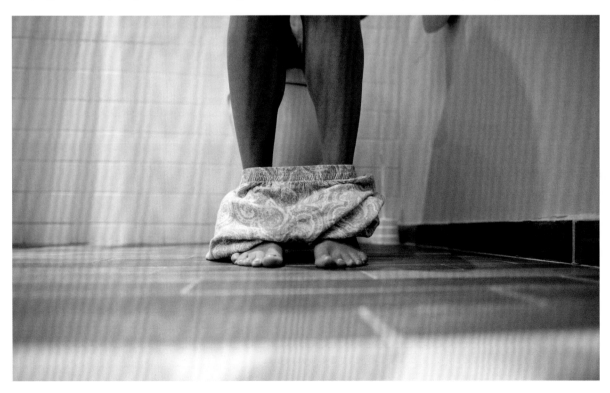

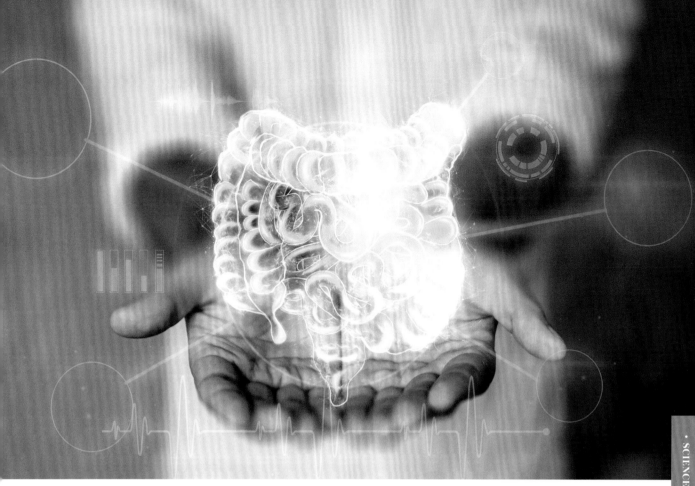

snacking throughout the day will prevent it from acting. This can lead to the growth of too much bacteria in the small intestine. So give your small intestine the time it needs to spruce itself up after eating before heading to the snack cupboard.

WE ARE LEGION

The large intestine is where our inside becomes a zoo. It contains literally billions of bacteria, the concentration increasing as it progresses towards the body's back door. The bacteria reside there, operating in what is normally a harmonious relationship with our body, team working in the breakdown of the remaining, more indigestible, parts of our diet. The large intestine is also important in ensuring that the liquid used in digestion is not needlessly excreted: ideally, enough should be reabsorbed to leave the faeces soft and smooth but not so much that it becomes hard lumps. Stress and illness can cause

'Stress and illness can cause the body to move the food along too quickly'

the body to move the food along too quickly, expelling faeces in a wet, diarrhoetic flood.

To extract every last morsel of nutrition from our food, the large intestine takes its time. Food meanders along, sometimes even backing up. The reason the large intestine always looks lumpy in illustrations is that the lumps are where the remaining food is kept, in bacteria-friendly bumps. A few times a day, the large intestine heaves the lump along, moving it closer to the exit. This is why doctors prescribe high-fibre foods for constipation: the fibre is very difficult for

the body to break down and it gives the muscles of the large intestine something to grab hold of when it next heaves the food along.

There's a wide variety in how long it takes food, or what's left of it, to go from mouth to bottom. For some people, it takes a day; for others it can be up to three and a half. Faster is not necessarily better; what counts is the consistency of what comes out the other end. A smooth, soft sausage, or a sausage with a few cracks are best according to the Bristol stool scale. This ranks poos from one to seven, with one being hard little lumps and seven a liquid with nothing solid. Type three (sausage with a few cracks) and type four (smooth, like toothpaste) are best. So if that's what you produce when you go to the loo, you don't need to worry about how long you're taking between poos: everything is moving along nicely down there. Give your gut a pat: it's doing its job, the silent partner in our body's daily routines.

Meet your microbiome

Your gut is home to thousands of microbial colonies, but most are there to help

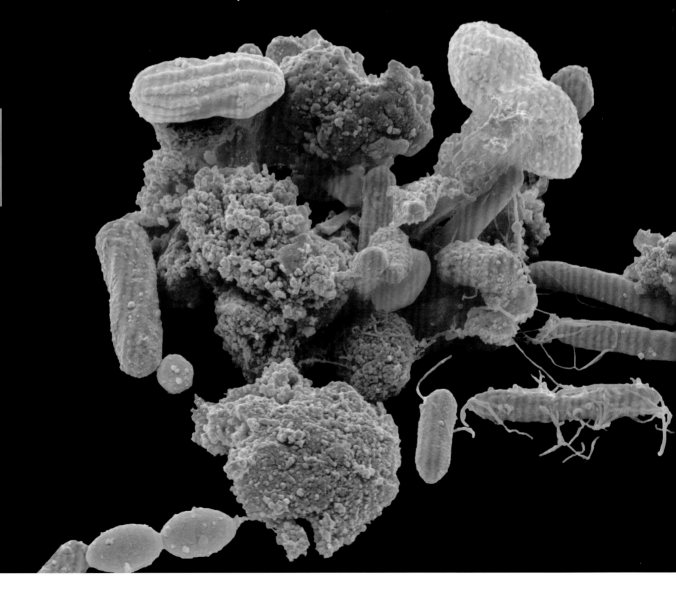

What do you perceive as being human? On a cellular level, you might be surprised to know that more than half of the cells in your body are non-human.

The collection of these cells, which make up about 57 per cent of your total cell count, is the microbiome. This contains an estimated 39 trillion microbes, living on or in human tissue. Despite its spectacular assortment of non-human cells, the microbiome is an essential part of being human, working to maintain good health and keep our human tissue thriving.

The kinds of cells that live in our microbiome include bacteria, fungi, parasites and viruses – and the largest number of these congregate in the gut. Here, these cells regulate the immune system, eliminate diseases and produce important vitamins.

WHAT IS A HEALTHY MICROBIOME?

In daily life, many people are unaware of the thousands of species that inhabit the body. In fact, being unaware of them is the first good sign of a healthy microbiome. This is because many of the microbes in the body are symbiotic, meaning that when working correctly, their presence allows both the human body and community of microorganisms to benefit.

Because microorganisms are invisible to the naked eye, we have limited control over the types of microbes that enter our bodies. A small number of those in the microbiome, known as pathogens, will be disease-causing. The body can remain healthy, even in the presence of pathogens, but there is a fine balance to be struck. If too many pathogens are introduced to the body, or an increased use of antibiotics lowers the number of helpful bacteria too much, the healthy microbiome is disturbed. This puts the body at a higher risk of developing disease.

THE MANY ROLES OF THE MICROBIOME

The microbiome has so many essential roles that it is often referred to as a 'supporting organ'. Two of its main functions are helping to keep the digestive system under control and assisting the immune system.

The mechanical digestion that human cells are responsible for can only do so much when it comes to completely breaking down our food. For many foods, we rely on gut bacteria. One example is polysaccharides – complex sugars that are found in plants. In the gut, bacteria produce the enzymes needed to digest polysaccharides. By breaking down these foods, the microbiome is responsible for turning food into its easily absorbed nutrients. These enzymes provide us with B vitamins, Vitamin K and short chain fatty acids. Without the microbiome to carry out this function, the nutritional value of food would be lowered.

When new organisms are introduced into the gut, and other regions of the body, the microbiome plays a key part in establishing which are safe and which to attack. This aspect of the immune system is essential as, without it, the aforementioned beneficial gut bacteria would be perceived as a threat and attacked by the body.

Microbes don't just fight dangerous cells after they enter the body. A layer of them, called a biofilm, serves as a protective shield on our skin against harmful bacteria and fungi. Similarly, in the gut, specific bacteria called Bifidobacteria prevent toxins from entering the bloodstream. Keeping toxins in the gut means they can soon be passed out of the body. However, if they were to travel through the intestinal wall and into the blood, toxins can wreak havoc as they spread fast in the bloodstream.

Microbiome activity in the gut also has the power to impact the mind, thanks to a nerve called the vagus nerve and the gut-brain axis. As microorganisms in the gut interact with the central nervous system, studies have shown that the brain's chemistry can be altered, impacting a person's mental health. This may even be able to influence a person's memory. Additionally, gut bacteria can even make you happier, as it is responsible for producing 95 per cent of

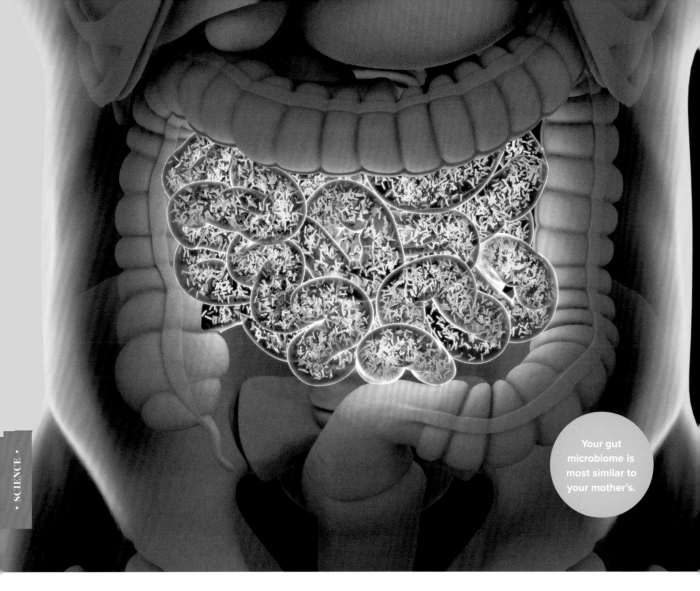

Your gut microbiome is most similar to your mother's.

the body's serotonin. This hormone is key in determining people's mental well-being as it stabilises mood.

CAN YOUR MICROBIOME CHANGE?

A person's microbiome is unique to them. At the beginning of life, its original makeup is determined by that of their mother. As a baby is born, its body is exposed to the microorganisms that exist in the mother's birth canal. Further significant additions to the microbiome are provided in milk during breastfeeding. These environmental impacts continue to occur throughout life. Microbiomes change based on events including (but not limited to) the food being eaten, medication taken, disease, exercise and age.

The more your microbiome changes, the better, according to research published in February 2021. Scientists discovered that people whose microbiome remained the same for long periods of their lives tend to die earlier than those whose microbial colonies varied over time. Generally, in the healthiest individuals studied, the microorganisms that were most prevalent during early adulthood became a smaller percentage of the gut microbiome over the following years. This enabled new species to grow in numbers in the body.

It isn't yet known whether people aged better as a result of the changed microbiome, or if it was the microbiome that adapted to the ageing body. However, research showed that the guts with the more transformed microbiome

appeared to be better suited to fighting chronic illness.

Transforming your gut microbiome is relatively easy to do. By drastically altering your diet, the levels of your body's bacteria species can change significantly in just four days. This trait is thought to have helped hunter gatherers, who could have had contrasting meals from day to day depending on available resources. With different gut bacteria being able to dominate the microbiome, more nutrients could be extracted from each varied food source.

HOW TO LOOK AFTER YOUR MICROBIOME

Our microbiomes may be personal to us, but one thing they all have in common is a huge variety of microorganisms that work to keep us alive and healthy. Some work to control fat storage, while others repair damaged gut lining or fight off harmful invading cells. The microbiome is almost like an army of workers with specialist skills, and when looking after it, this might be a useful way to imagine it.

To keep the microbiome working well, a huge combination of workers are needed to keep the body in check. There are many steps that can be taken to maximise our healthy gut flora. We are often told to eat a lot of fruit and vegetables, but eating a variety of these is better for the microbiome. Each contains different chemicals that can help particular microbes.

Feeding the gut is essential, but so is allowing it to rest. By avoiding snacking, your microbiome isn't overworked. Additionally, instead of feeding existing microbes, you can consume live ones. Yoghurt, kimchi and other fermented products are good for this. Meanwhile, consuming alcohol in moderation creates a diverse microbiome, but too much will have the opposite effect.

WHEN IS A FAECAL TRANSPLANT NEEDED?

In some instances, such as the overuse of antibiotics, the levels of 'good' bacteria become so low that they are significantly outnumbered by pathogenic cells. When immediate alterations to the microbiome are required to restore a patient to health, microbes can be transplanted from a donor.

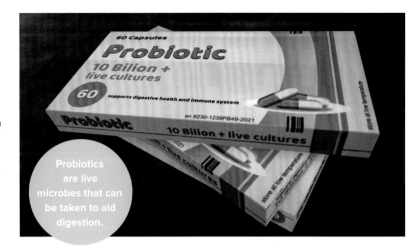

Probiotics are live microbes that can be taken to aid digestion.

Faecal transplantation is usually carried out by colonoscopy and involves adding faecal bacteria from another person directly into the recipient's colon. This donor's microbiome is analysed before the procedure to make sure they are healthy and that the transplant will cure the bacterial imbalance.

WHAT IS THE HUMAN MICROBIOME PROJECT?

There is so much left to learn about the microbiome. It makes up around two per cent of the human body's mass and many scientists compare its importance to that of vital organs. One initiative that has greatly improved our knowledge of the microbiome is the Human Microbiome Project, which was launched by the US National Institutes of Health in 2007. The project funds research into both the

human and non-human cells of the body, with the goal to better understand the microbiome. The primary focus of the Human Microbiome Project was to study these cells' contribution to health and disease.

Scientists are working to map the microbiome, as a major indicator of health, to gain understanding of how these cells impact nutrition, immunity and disease in the gut and other ecosystems of the body.

Over the last few decades, scientists have developed a relatively good understanding of the general importance of the microbiome, but know less about individual species and their roles. One way that these are now being studied is by using artificial intelligence alongside data from genetic sequencing. When combined, the machine learning algorithms can highlight recurring patterns in DNA to explore which cells usually exist together in the microbiome.

Thanks to ongoing research, thousands of unknown bacteria, viruses and other microbes have been discovered in the human gut. In single studies, thousands of links between specific species and chronic diseases have been made. As our knowledge of this extensive and complex microbial community expands, drug treatment for some of the most debilitating gut diseases can be improved and we can better assist our microbiomes in continuing to assist us.

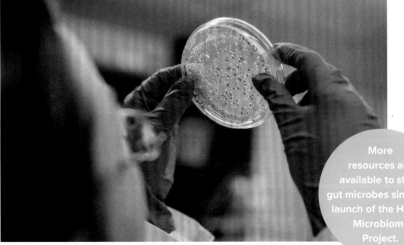

More resources are available to study gut microbes since the launch of the Human Microbiome Project.

Signs of an unhealthy GUT

We rely on the digestive tract to deliver nutrients, but what happens when its function is altered?

By looking at any recent diagram of the digestive system, it appears to be little more than one long, winding tube. Its general role is to carry ingested material – of varying composition – from mouth to anus, before its waste products are released from the body.

While these anatomical diagrams are effective at highlighting the route that food and liquid takes, they can provide a deceivingly simplified representation of the process. In actuality, there are intricate microscopic details hidden within every section of the gut, and complex mechanics that manipulate food and its nutrients to benefit the body. These are the steps that are continually being performed inside a healthy gut without being noticed – that is, until a healthy gut becomes decidedly unhealthy.

When someone suffers from a gastrointestinal disease or condition, difficulties are added to daily life. These range from not being able to eat certain foods (and the added worry that surrounds mealtimes as a result) to experiencing constant pain and many hours in the bathroom.

For each intestinal illness, the levels of severity can vary. But those who haven't been diagnosed with a specific illness are not immune to an unhealthy gut by any means. Many gastrointestinal issues are temporary and require less treatment.

Stomach pains can be caused by a variety of events, from food poisoning to stress. Because discomfort in the abdomen is a symptom shared by so many diseases, and other biological events, it can be hard to recognise signs of a specific condition. The best thing to do when suffering from regular or persistent abdominal pain is to consult a medical professional. This stops some of the more serious causes being left untreated.

Coeliac disease

The gut's gluten retaliation

For some people, food products such as bread, pasta and cakes trigger an autoimmune response in the gut. This is because their body mistakenly perceives gluten to be a threat. Gluten is the general name for the proteins found in wheat and, unfortunately for those with coeliac disease, it is present in many foods.

When launching into the autoimmune response, cells attack the gluten. Instead of saving the body from true danger (as the immune system usually does), the reaction to what should be harmless cells causes unnecessary damage to the small intestine. As the intestine becomes inflamed, the large surface area of the small intestine is reduced, limiting the water and nutrients that can be absorbed through the intestine's tissue. As a result, symptoms of coeliac disease include malnutrition – from the lack of nutrient absorption out of the intestine – stomach pains and diarrhoea from the limited water being transported out of the gut.

Around one per cent of the population suffer from coeliac disease and the only effective treatment is to follow a gluten-free diet. Continuing to consume gluten in the long term can lead to the development of other autoimmune diseases and neurological issues such as epilepsy. Today, there are many gluten-free alternatives in restaurants and supermarkets.

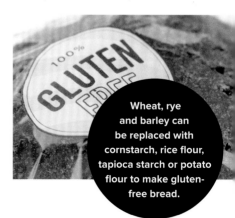

Wheat, rye and barley can be replaced with cornstarch, rice flour, tapioca starch or potato flour to make gluten-free bread.

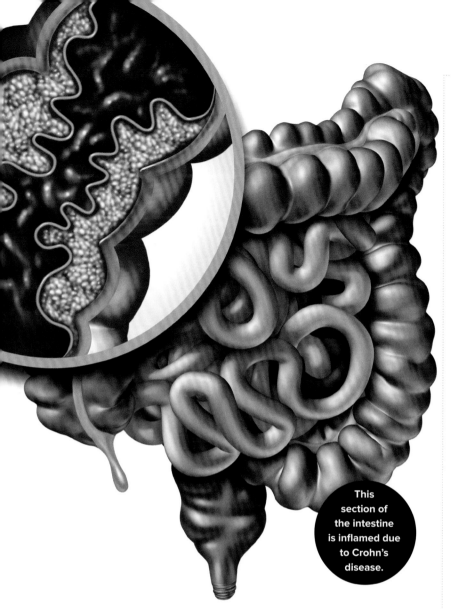

This section of the intestine is inflamed due to Crohn's disease.

Gastroesophageal reflux disease (GERD)

The stomach's destructive power

When you eat a meal, food travels through the digestive system, being passed between organs as it is churned and broken down. Inside the stomach, strong acids and enzymes work to release the nutrients from food that the body requires. In order to prevent the stomach from digesting itself, a mucus barrier is constantly created to line it. Not all of our innards are quite so hardy, and the oesophagus is one of those. The oesophagus is the tube that connects our throats to our stomachs. To separate this vertical passage from the acidic contents of our stomachs, a ring of muscle called the lower oesophageal sphincter remains contracted and closed. It opens to allow food to enter the stomach, and usually stops stomach contents entering the oesophagus. GERD symptoms are caused when this muscle is weak or relaxes when it shouldn't. Without a barrier, stomach contents flow into the oesophagus and can irritate its cells.

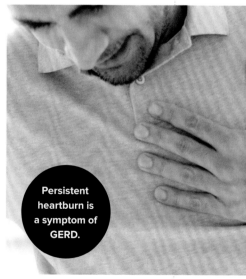

Persistent heartburn is a symptom of GERD.

Crohn's

Intestinal inflammation can cause unwelcome flare-ups

Crohn's is a bowel disease that inflames the digestive tract, causing stomach pain, fatigue, diarrhoea and blood in faeces. These symptoms usually arise during childhood or early in adulthood, but the exact cause of Crohn's disease isn't known. The chronic disease is thought to be genetic, as 15 per cent of sufferers have a close relative with Crohn's. Usually, it targets the small intestine and the beginning of the large intestine, but it's possible for Crohn's to affect any part of the digestive tract.

One of the difficulties faced by those with the disease is not knowing when a debilitating flare-up is going to arise. With little warning, symptoms can escalate to induce greater abdominal pain and urgent bowel movements. For this period, sufferers may lose their appetite, feel drained of energy and lose significant weight. Anti-inflammatory medication is prescribed to Crohn's sufferers, which helps to manage bowel movements and enable some people to feel well for weeks or months at a time.

Colitis

Complications in the colon

When inflammation occurs in the large intestine, this is colitis. One form of colitis, called ulcerative colitis, is the second of the two inflammatory bowel diseases. This type is similar to Crohn's disease but is limited to the large intestine. In the worst cases of inflammation, sections of the large intestine need to be removed in surgery.

Another form, known as Pseudomembranous colitis, is caused by the accumulation of the bacteria Clostridium difficile (C. diff). This bacteria is naturally found living in the intestines, but when too much healthy bacteria is killed off, C. diff can build up and release too many inflammation-inducing toxins.

Like the majority of the body, the colon relies on a healthy blood flow. In an instance whereby a clot greatly reduces blood flow to the colon, ischemic colitis can arise. The lack of nutrient-carrying blood to the intestine can leave its lining damaged with bleeding sores.

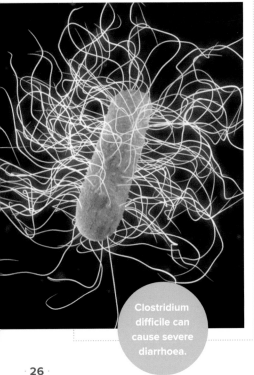

Clostridium difficile can cause severe diarrhoea.

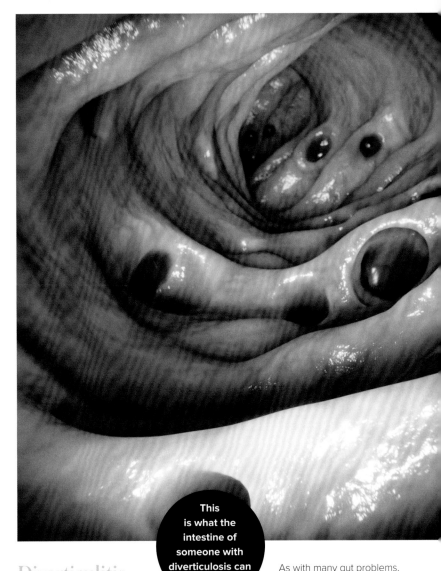

This is what the intestine of someone with diverticulosis can look like.

Diverticulitis

What causes painful pouches in the colon?

As we age, parts of our body can get weaker, and the gut is no exception. When the colon develops naturally weaker areas, small sections of it can give way under pressure and form little pouches in the colon wall. These pouches – called diverticula – are usually only marble-sized, but can easily tear and become infected. Someone who has diverticula, which can exist harmlessly in the intestine, has diverticulosis, while the infection and inflammation of the pouches is called diverticulitis.

As with many gut problems, the level of severity and impact on quality of life can vary greatly. Some of the worst of this pain is caused by significant bowel ruptures. Doctors administer antibiotics for some diverticula infections, or they may suggest specific diets that reduce the risk of inflammation.

This treatment can be essential, as leaving diverticulitis untreated can make it much worse. Pus can collect in abscesses near the area of infection after a while. If these make their way through the wall of the intestine, it can cause life-threatening infections. Additionally, if diverticula tear too much, scarring can block the intestine and prevent it from carrying out its function.

Peptic ulcer disease

A defenceless stomach can result in sores

As its name implies, this disease is caused by peptic ulcers that form in the stomach and the upper areas of the small intestine. These painful sores appear when acid in the stomach wears away the inner walls of the gut, to create a burning and bloated sensation in the stomach. In a healthy gut, the mucus layer that lines the stomach and intestines protects this sort of damage by acid. However, it is a fine balance. If the volume of mucus in the stomach decreases, or too much acid forms, this barrier stops doing its job.

One of the most common causes of these ulcers is the presence of the bacteria Heliobacter pylori. This bacteria may be passed between people by close contact or may enter the body in food and drink. Infection by this bacteria doesn't necessarily mean that the stomach will suffer. Sometimes the bacteria lives in mucus in the digestive tract without causing injury.

The constant use of anti-inflammatory medication, such as ibuprofen can also increase the likelihood of peptic ulcer disease. As ibuprofen prevents inflammation, it also reduces hormones called prostaglandins from being produced. These are lipid hormones, which gather at areas of inflammation to protect tissue. As ibuprofen and other similar medications reduce inflammation without producing this protective barrier, the stomach walls become more vulnerable to acid over time.

Peptic ulcers can make people feel sick and not want to eat.

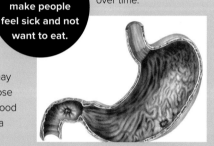

Irritable bowel syndrome (IBS)

What happens when gut-brain interactions are disrupted?

Did you know that your intestines and emotional areas of the brain are connected? This means that emotions can have a direct impact on gut health. The symptoms of IBS, for example, can become heightened by feelings of stress and anxiety, which release chemicals in the brain that impact the intestines and how the feeling of digestion is portrayed. For those with IBS, nerves in the gut can be oversensitive. Small amounts of gas, that would normally cause little discomfort, result in bloating, diarrhoea, constipation and strong pain in the stomach, which usually eases after going to the toilet.

IBS is common and can affect people for days, weeks or months at a time. While there's no 'one-diet-fits-all' cure, most people find that eating fresh foods without incorporating too much fresh fruit, relieves symptoms. Fatty and spicy foods can make IBS worse, along with skipping meals. Keeping a food diary can help to find out which foods are best for your body.

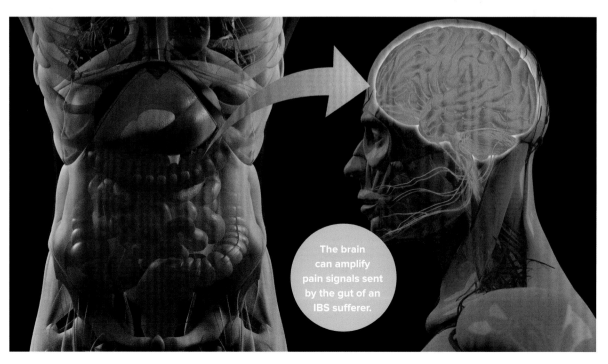

The brain can amplify pain signals sent by the gut of an IBS sufferer.

Healthy gut, happy you

Discover ten ways you can improve your health and make your life better

The gut is a generally unassuming part of the body that takes all we drop into it and gets on with its business. But there are some things you can do to keep it happy and thus the rest of your body happy, too. Some are quite obvious but always worth restating, others less clear but still worth doing. Here, we go through some of the ways to keep things moving down below.

Eat the rainbow

Why eating lots of colourful food is good for the body as well as pleasing to the eye

Red strawberries, green cabbage, blue, er, blueberries, yellow bananas and orange, yes, oranges. Natural foods are a riot of colour and flavours. Many of the specific chemicals that give fruit and vegetables their distinctive colours have been found to have health benefits, while simply adding greater variety to our diets is good. We are descendants of hunter gatherers who usually ate up to 500 different plants in their diets. Eating the rainbow is an attempt to regain some of that variety.

Lycopene, which makes cherries and other fruit red, has antioxidant properties while also reducing blood pressure and cholesterol. The carotenoids alpha-

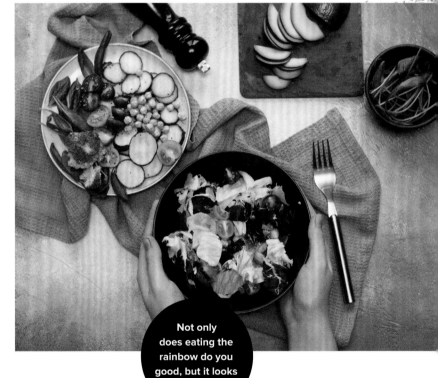

Not only does eating the rainbow do you good, but it looks wonderful.

carotene and beta-carotene, which produce orange and yellow fruit and vegetables, have been linked to reduced risks of heart attacks and cancer, although the specific evidence is not strong. Greenness comes from chlorophyll, but green vegetables have many other useful chemicals. In particular, broccoli, cabbage, Brussels sprouts and kale are rich in sulphur, a trace chemical

that is important to human health but not readily available outside these leafy greens. Purple foods such as aubergines and beetroot contain nitrates, which may help in reducing your blood pressure.

Rather than seeking specific health improvements attached to each colour, eating the rainbow is better seen as a reminder to eat a variety of foods: the greatest benefit lies in that very variety.

> **Green tea is rich in polyphenols and it's good to drink, too.**

Eat less meat

Should we cut down on the amount of meat we eat?

Human beings are omnivores. That we can eat almost everything is the result of our long past as hunter gatherers. But studies of modern-day hunter gatherers have shown that, for most of the year, they were gatherers more than hunters.

Coming closer to the present, the Mediterranean diet, which has proven benefits, features less meat than modern Western diets. Specific research on reducing meat consumption has shown that doing so results in a string of health benefits including lower risk of heart disease, strokes, lower blood pressure, lower cholesterol, and less chance of obesity and some cancers. In particular, eating a lot of meat high in saturated fats — sausages, bacon — tends to go with increased risk of obesity and all its associated morbidities.

It's not really hard to work out: highly processed meat is not as good for you as less processed meat, something that applies just as much to processed plant-based foods. Buying fresh food and cooking it yourself is always far better than slapping a pre-made meal in the microwave.

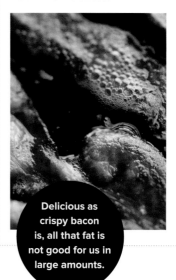

> **Delicious as crispy bacon is, all that fat is not good for us in large amounts.**

Eat more polyphenols

Good news: not all your favourite foods are bad for you

For those who find the puritanical finger wagging of nutritionists depressing, the discovery of the beneficial effects of polyphenols has been a godsend. Eating a diet rich in them has been shown to reduce the risk of developing chronic disease, such as diabetes and heart problems.

Among the common diet items containing polyphenols are tea, cocoa, broad beans and apples, which have flavanols; citrus fruit has flavanones; coffee has hydroxycinnamates, as do many fruits; apples, tea and onions have flavanols; while red wine is rich in resveratrol. Researchers have not yet established exactly how polyphenols work to benefit us, but their discovery has come as a welcome boon to those wanting to eat and drink some of the good things in life with a clear conscience.

So, coffee, tea, red wine, chocolate. Anyone would be happy with these in a diet. But, as always, to keep the gut truly happy, even foods stuffed full with polyphenols have to be eaten in balance with the rest of our diet.

Eat more fibre

How come eating more of what we can't digest is so important for our health?

If the gut is all about extracting every last bit of nourishment from the food we eat, it might seem surprising that one of the best things we can do to improve the health of the gut is to eat more food containing stuff that the gut can't digest: fibre.

Fibre is the parts of plants, vegetables, nuts and roots that our stomachs can't break down in the small intestine. Instead, they get passed on to the large intestine. In distinction to the quick-working small intestine, the large intestine takes its time, holding parcels of undigested food in pockets while the innumerable bacteria that live there get to work on the fibre.

The short-chain fatty acids that the microbes split some of the fibre into help insulin sensitivity and reduce the levels of glucose and lipids in the blood, which indirectly protects against cardiovascular disease, obesity and diabetes. Then, when the bacteria have finished, the remaining fibres gives the lower intestine something to grab hold of when it has to push what's left further along. Fibres also absorb some water, which helps when it comes to pushing out what's left at the end of the gut, stopping constipation and making going to the toilet less of a strain. Rough fibre in, softer poo out.

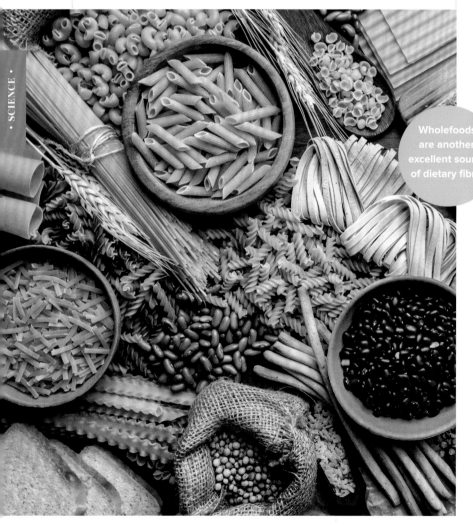

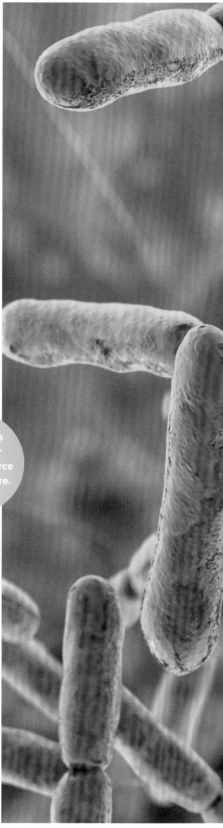

Wholefoods are another excellent source of dietary fibre.

SCIENCE

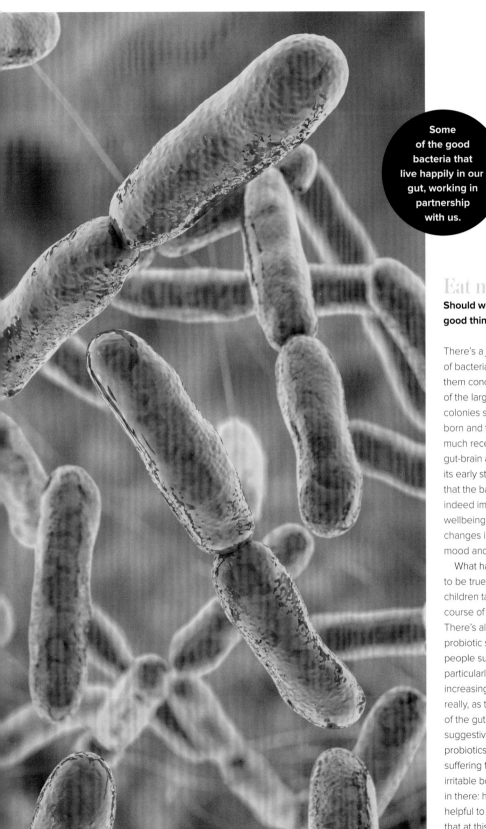

Eat more bacteria

Should we add bacteria to our list of good things to eat?

There's a jungle inside us. Literally trillions of bacteria live in our gut, with most of them concentrated in the lower reaches of the large intestine. These bacterial colonies start forming the moment we are born and they have become the focus of much recent research looking at the gut-brain axis. While the research is still in its early stages, tentative findings show that the balance of bacteria in our gut is indeed important to our health and wellbeing, with some studies even linking changes in the gut flora to changes in mood and anxiety levels.

What has been shown, quite robustly, to be true, is the beneficial effects of children taking probiotic supplements if a course of antibiotics is causing diarrhoea. There's also reliable data saying that probiotic supplements can be useful to people suffering from constipation, particularly when combined with increasing fibre intake (not surprising, really, as the fibre provides food for some of the gut bacteria). Less robust, but suggestive, research has found that probiotics can be helpful to people suffering from Crohn's disease and irritable bowel syndrome. There's a jungle in there: helping it grow might well be helpful to you (but we can't say more than that at this stage).

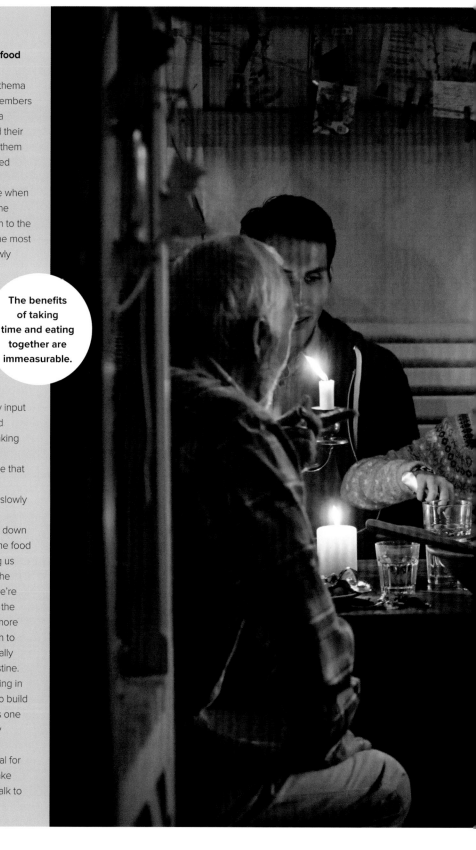

Eat slow
Take your time and enjoy your food

The very idea of fast food is anathema to many cultures. The writer remembers an Italian restauranteur ejecting a German couple who complained their food was taking too long, telling them to go to McDonald's if they wanted fast food.

The benefits of taking our time when eating are varied, running from the physical, through the social, even to the spiritual, but we will begin with the most obvious benefit. Food eaten slowly tastes better. And the curious paradox of better-tasting food is that we don't eat as much of it.

In part, that's because taking time to eat gives our gut the chance to signal to the brain that it's had enough, but it's also a consequence of a richer sensory input from the food itself. Eating should encompass all the senses and taking time allows this to happen — and therefore cues the brain to realise that it has had enough.

On the level of the gut, eating slowly helps with digestion, allowing everything to run more smoothly down there. Chewing more prepares the food for the stomach, as well as giving us more opportunity to appreciate the flavour and texture of the food we're eating in the moment, and when the food arrives in the stomach it is more spaced out, allowing the stomach to sort through it better before it finally gets passed on to the small intestine.

On the social level, slower eating in company gives the opportunity to build social relationships, and if there's one thing research has unequivocally demonstrated, it's that social relationships are hugely beneficial for every aspect of our health. So, take your time, enjoy your food, and talk to each other while you do it.

The benefits of taking time and eating together are immeasurable.

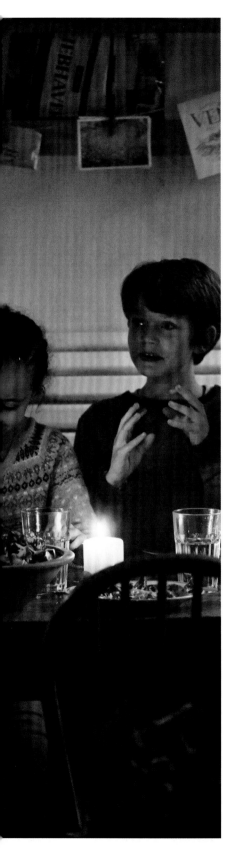

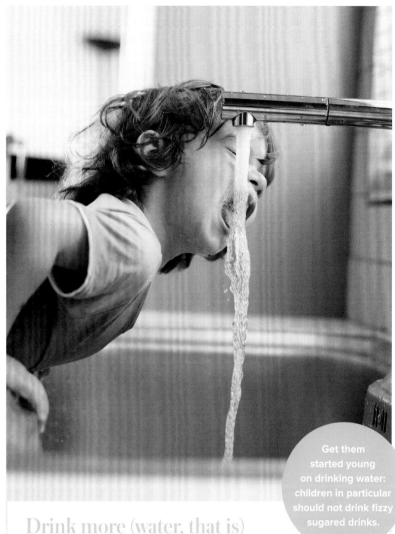

Get them started young on drinking water: children in particular should not drink fizzy sugared drinks.

Drink more (water, that is)

Adam's ale is still the best way of drinking

Our bodies are 60 per cent water, so it should come as no surprise that we need liquid to keep us alive. Indeed, we will die much more quickly from thirst than from hunger, although the exact time varies considerably according to the conditions (hot and dry is worse than cool).

The National Academy of Medicine recommends men take 12.5 cups of liquid a day, women nine cups, pregnant women ten cups and breastfeeding women 13 cups. All this water is required to maintain the body's homeostasis, the balance between water gained and lost during the course of our normal activities. The brain monitors water levels constantly, adjusting them to cope with what we are doing, whether it be sitting down in a cool room or running under the hot sun.

With respect to the gut, not drinking enough water often contributes towards constipation. If the body is not getting enough water, it will reabsorb fluid as it passes through the large intestine, making the faeces drier, harder and less easy to pass. As an easy step towards better gut health, drinking more water ranks high.

Drink less

A bit of a no-brainer here: too much alcohol is bad for us

The more difficult question to answer for sure is whether a moderate level of drinking can have some health benefits. Studies comparing the health effects of not drinking alcohol at all when compared to drinking moderate amounts, that is not more than one alcoholic drink a day, are mixed, with some showing health benefits in not drinking at all while others seem to show that moderate drinking can be beneficial to health.

Given that these studies have conflicting findings, and that the health benefits one way or the other are not great, the common-sense approach is that while heavy drinking has demonstrable and major ill effects on health, there is little to choose between total abstinence and modest amounts of alcohol. Given its place as a social lubricant and, for many people, part of the good life, drinking in moderation is a perfectly rational choice to make given the state of the research at present. Cheers!

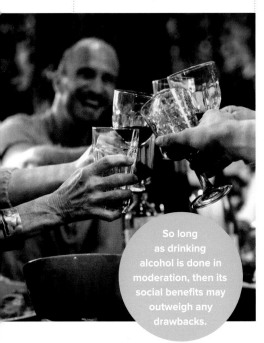

So long as drinking alcohol is done in moderation, then its social benefits may outweigh any drawbacks.

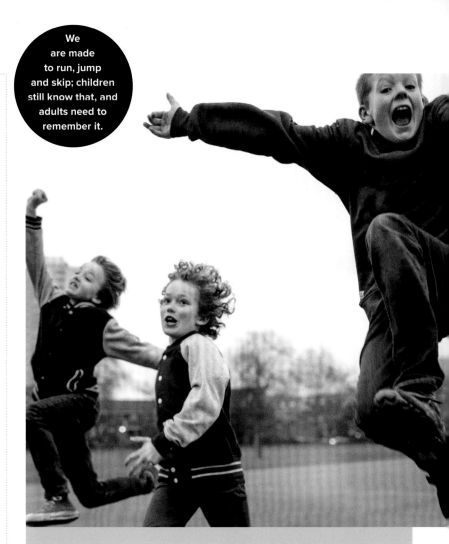

We are made to run, jump and skip; children still know that, and adults need to remember it.

This body was made for walking

Why exercise is one of the best things we can do for our health

300,000 years of history have fitted us for movement. Indeed, even before modern Homo sapiens evolved, we developed for a life of constant movement: there is no other animal on Earth that can run for as long or as far as humans. We lost our fur and began to sweat so that the body could stop itself overheating when running for mile after mile.

Research has demonstrated the overwhelming benefits of regular exercise. Indeed, if it was a medicine, it would be hailed as a miracle cure, helping almost every facet of our health and wellbeing. Indeed, it would be easier to draw up a list of what exercise doesn't help than what it does help. But to take some obvious examples, people who exercise regularly have a 30 per cent lower risk of early death, and lower incidences of a range of chronic diseases and mental illnesses, including heart disease, diabetes, strokes, breast cancer, bowel cancer, osteoarthritis, hip fractures, dementia, depression and chronic stress.

For exercise to truly be exercise, it needs to raise the heart and breathing rate, so medium to brisk walking is enough to have all these benefits, not to mention more vigorous activities that may be even more helpful. Best of all is to increase everyday activity, like taking the stairs rather than using a lift, and walking to work rather than catching a bus.

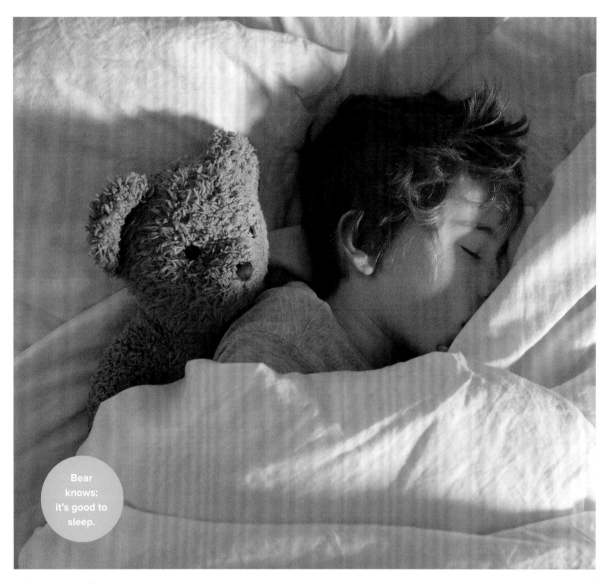

Bear knows: it's good to sleep.

Sleep well

Enough sleep is as important to health as good food and exercise

A healthy lifestyle has three strands: good food, exercise and sleep. It might be hard to believe, but getting eight hours of sleep a night is as beneficial for your health as exercise and a good diet. Sleep, rather than being a non-productive down time, is the period when the body sets itself to right and depriving the body of adequate amounts of sleep leads to major long-term consequences in ill health. One of the most counter-intuitive findings is that sleeping more helps people stay slim. The reasons why are

complex and little understood, but the findings are clear. One consequence of better sleep is that people eat less when they are awake. As with exercise, a lifetime of good nights' sleep has huge health benefits, reducing the risk of almost all the major chronic diseases of the modern world, including heart disease, strokes and diabetes. The immune system also benefits from the body's rest: one study found people who were sleep deprived were nearly three times as likely to catch cold when compared to those who got eight hours a night. Sleep also helps mental health: people who suffer from reduced or

disturbed sleep patterns are more likely to develop depression than regular eight-hour sleepers. So, sweet dreams of good health.

'People who were sleep deprived were nearly three times as likely to catch a cold'

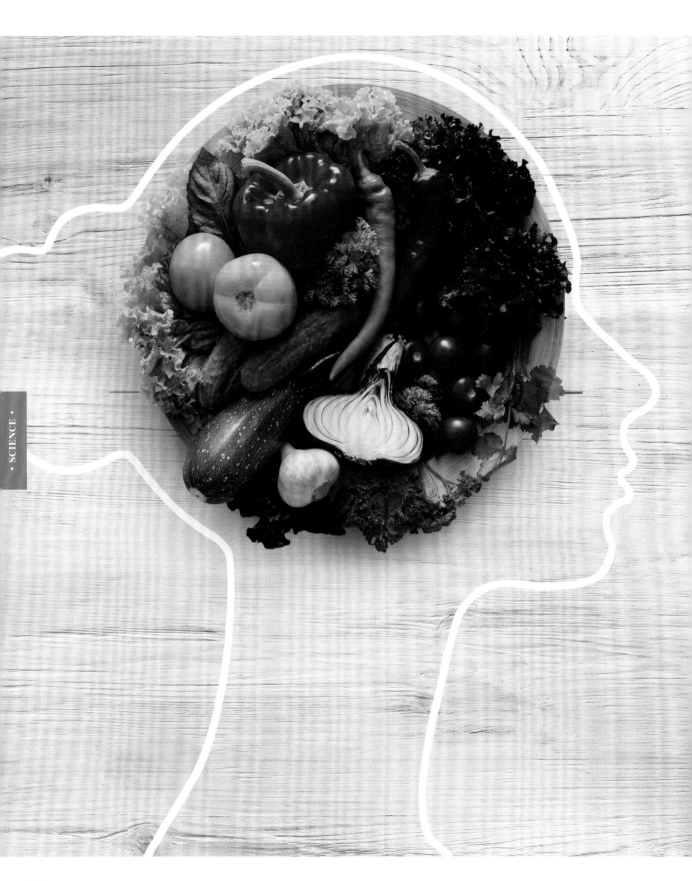

The gut-brain AXIS

How our brain talks to our gut and how
our gut answers back to the brain

Having finished a good meal and sat back in your chair, do you then direct your intention inwards and issue instructions to your gut to get on with the job of digesting? Obviously not. Still less do you have to tell the stomach to start with the liquid and then move on to churning the food by retropulsion. The stomach, along with the rest of the gut, simply gets on with the job.

THE ENTERIC NERVOUS SYSTEM

The gut can do its job, quietly and normally with very little fuss, because it is controlled and communicates via an entirely separate signalling system to the one we use to control our movements and direct our thoughts. That one is the central nervous system, starting at the brain and going down through the spine before radiating out to all our muscles.

The gut operates under a different system: the enteric nervous system. This is what communicates between the different sections of the gut, telling the small intestine to get a move on as a fresh batch of food is coming into the stomach or asking the large intestine to draw some more fluid from the fibrous mass its working on.

The enteric nervous system is set into the gut's lining and it is composed of 500 million neurons, which is ten times as many as the spinal cord (although only 0.5 per cent of the mind-boggling 86 billion neurons in the brain). It communicates with the other nervous systems in the body via the vagus nerve and prevertebral ganglia. After all, the brain does need to know if we haven't eaten for three days or if we're so full that even the normally hyperstretchy stomach really can't fit any more food in.

However, the extraordinary result of experimental studies is that the enteric nervous system is perfectly happy to go on functioning even if its connection to the vagus nerve is cut. It's no wonder it's sometimes called our second brain. It needs to be. There's a lot going on inside us that it has to look after.

THE JUNGLE INSIDE

One of the key areas the enteric nervous system has to monitor is the veritable ecosystem of life that exists in our gut, particularly the latter section of the large intestine. The gut contains truly mind-boggling numbers of bacteria: ten to the power of 14 (that is a one followed by 14 noughts). That's ten times more microbes than there are cells in the human body. So only one in ten of the cells in our body are actually us: we play host to colonies of bacteria that vastly outnumber us. We are only at the start of investigating the effect of our internal jungle on our bodies and minds, but how did all these microbes get there in the first place?

For the first nine months of life, a baby exists in the only truly sterile environment it will ever know. In the womb, the baby is protected from the outside world. But all this changes from birth. Emerging through the birth canal, the baby comes into the world with its first colonists: passengers picked up from the mother's vaginal flora, bacteria it came into contact with from its mother with the mother's first embrace. This first colonisation is incredibly swift: some bacteria can produce their next generation in 20 minutes. By the time the baby is safe in its mother's arms, her parting gift, her own unique mix of bacteria, will be busily establishing themselves within the little suckling baby. Breastfeeding and normal motherly contact also help to establish a good mix of bacteria in the new baby. Although the initial colonisation is very swift, it's usually three years before the flora of the gut settle down into comfortable equilibrium.

These rapidly expanding colonies of bacteria in our gut play an essential, although not yet well understood, role in the development of both the central and enteric nervous systems in the weeks following birth. What's more, as the immune system lining the gut interacts with the microbiota living in the gut, it learns quickly and thoroughly how to distinguish between good, neutral and bad bacteria: the immune system learns and its single most important learning aid is the bacteria living in our gut.

WHAT'S INSIDE AFFECTS WHAT'S OUTSIDE

The vagus nerve is the longest nerve in our body, starting from the brain stem and going down to the gut, while also monitoring the heart, lungs and other internal organs. The enteric nervous system sends it information concerning what is going on in the gut, and it returns information to the gut, in particular about our stress levels. So there is a very good reason that we feel nerves – that is, stress – in our stomach region. Under stress, the brain is sending messages, via the vagus nerve, to the gut to prepare for possible emergency action.

A nervous system honed on the plains of Africa, sensing danger, tells the gut to get on with things: diarrhoea as the result of stress is the body responding to an evolutionary imperative to be ready to run for our lives. But nowadays, not many of us have to run from hunting lions. Stress, the marker of danger, for too many of us is in danger of becoming generalised as a response to the strains of everyday life.

INFLAMMATORY STRESS

The immune system has a difficult job. Sometimes, if it becomes too active, it can lead to the body being in a permanent state of low-level inflammation. As a chronic condition, low-level inflammation appears to be connected with a wide variety of disorders, including Alzheimer's and depression. One of the ways this happens is that chronic stress produces leaky gut syndrome, leading to some of our gut flora passing out of the gut, where they should be, into the bloodstream, where they shouldn't.

A number of studies have now shown that clinical depression is often linked with chronic low-level inflammation. So given that inflammation is often a result of imbalances in the gut flora, leading to leaky gut syndrome, some researchers have started investigating to see if restoring a better balance to the bacteria within our gut can help to improve our overall mood. A Dutch team, working with a group of volunteers, fed them helpful bacteria (apart from the control group, who were given a placebo) and monitored their answers to a set of questions measuring anger, brooding and despair. Over the four-week study, the group who were given the bacteria mix showed a ten per cent improvement in their feelings, particularly with respect to anger and brooding, when compared to the control group.

A ten per cent improvement is not huge, but it is past the point of coincidence. While psychiatric drugs produce much bigger changes, they often produce major side effects. The daily

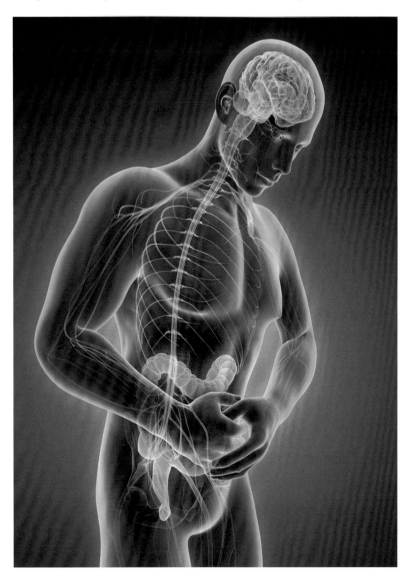

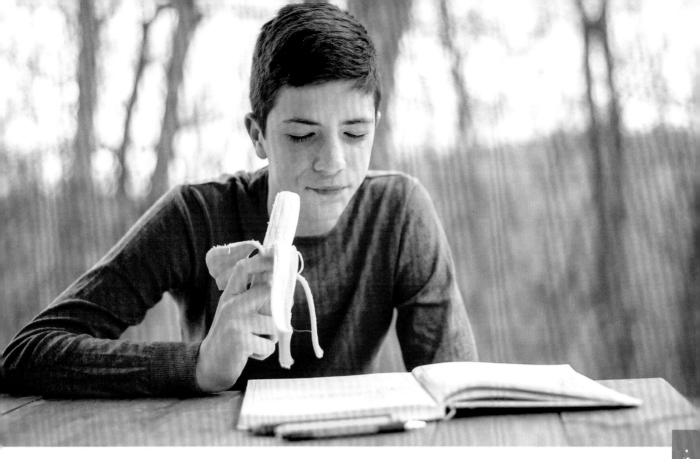

dose of bacteria had no obvious drawbacks. So it appears that changing the mix of bacteria in our gut can change the way we feel. At this point, it is beginning to seem that the body might better be described as a Commonwealth than a single organism.

MANAGING STRESS

If changing the mix of our gut bacteria can improve mood, can it also do something to improve the chronic levels of stress many of us experience? For while stress can be caused by leaky gut syndrome, in today's world it's just as likely to come from external factors that we cannot control such as work, family and money worries. While we may not be able to control how many deadlines we have, the health of our mum and dad or the cost of living, perhaps we can do something about how we experience this stress.

One study showed that ingesting a daily amount of Bifidobacterium bifidum reduced the subjective feelings of stress experienced by the experimental subjects. Following on from that finding, a

'Clinical depression is often linked with chronic low-level inflammation'

further eight-week study fed subjects either Bifidobacterium longum 1714 or a placebo, while measuring the subjects' experience of day-to-day stress. The subjects fed the bacteria reported, and were measured via a series of tests, to have experienced a 15 per cent reduction in their feelings of stress at the end of the study.

Although the tests to measure stress had not changed – plunging a hand into ice-cold water for as long as the subject could bear it – the people who had taken the bacteria had lower levels of stress hormones than before they had started taking it. Other tests also showed an

improvement in the subjects' performance in memory tasks – remember that stress is associated with the development of diseases such as Alzheimer's.

Early studies have also begun to see whether improving the balance of intestinal flora could help with depression. Studies with mice have indicated that gut bacteria can help mice that have been manipulated to suffer from depression-like symptoms. With findings linking depression to low-level inflammation, a rich vein of new research is opening up, one that might produce valuable help for one of the most common mental-health problems today.

So, we have to ask ourselves, is the cure in our gut? The honest answer is probably not. But by ensuring a healthier balance within us, it seems that we will be able to achieve a healthier balance with respect to the outside world, too. It looks like we should be cultivating the jungle within. The old saying was that the path to a man's heart led through his stomach. It now appears that, for all of us, the path through the gut takes us to better health.

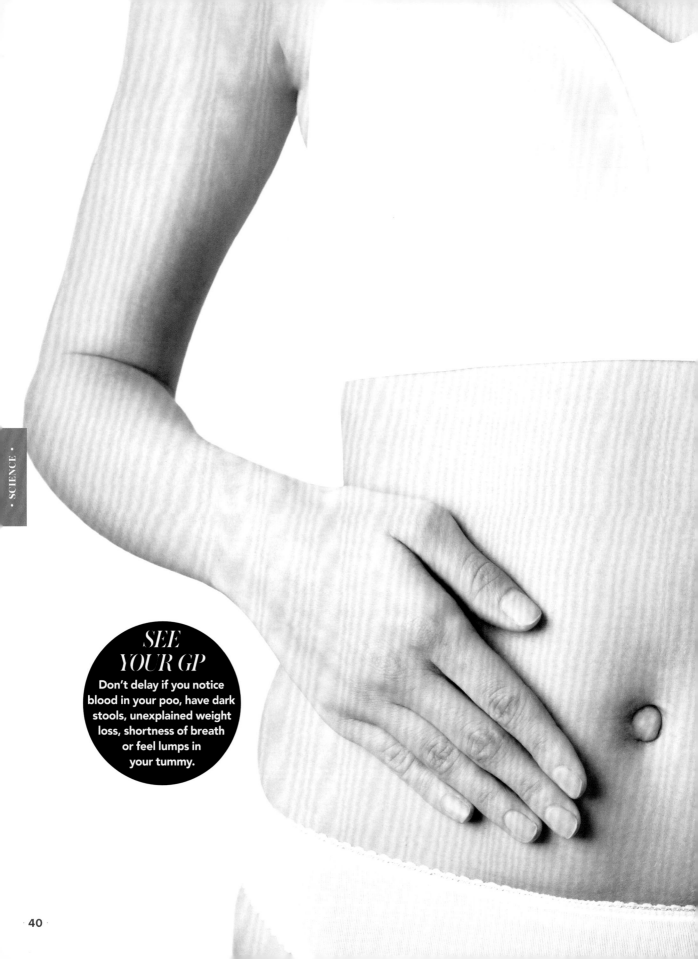

SEE YOUR GP

Don't delay if you notice blood in your poo, have dark stools, unexplained weight loss, shortness of breath or feel lumps in your tummy.

What's your GUT telling you?

If you're suffering with tummy troubles, take our test to find a fix

There's a complex connection between the digestive system and overall health – and if it's out of whack, it will impact elsewhere in the body. Your gut is home to trillions of bacteria, known as the gut microbiome and is responsible for the absorption of essential nutrients to aid the immune system, give us energy and boost brain function. So if things aren't feeling great in the digestion department, use the flow chart to discover the reason for your tummy troubles – and sort it with our expert's advice.

41

FOLLOW THE FLOWCHART

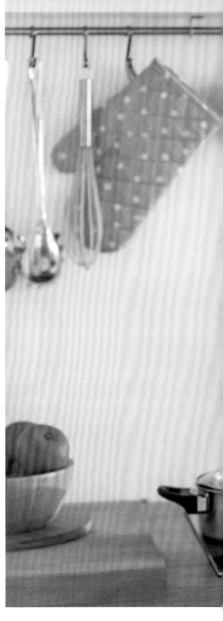

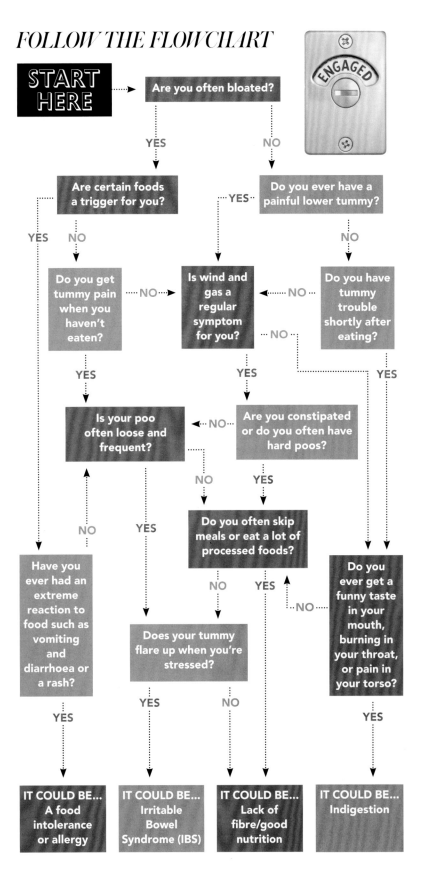

START HERE → Are you often bloated?

Are you often bloated?
- YES ↓
- NO ↓

YES branch: Are certain foods a trigger for you?
- YES →
- NO ↓

NO branch: Do you ever have a painful lower tummy?
- YES →
- NO ↓

Are certain foods a trigger for you?
- YES ↓
- NO → Do you get tummy pain when you haven't eaten?

Do you get tummy pain when you haven't eaten?
- NO → Is wind and gas a regular symptom for you?
- YES ↓

Do you ever have a painful lower tummy? → YES → Is wind and gas a regular symptom for you?

Do you have tummy trouble shortly after eating?
- NO → Is wind and gas a regular symptom for you?
- YES ↓

Is wind and gas a regular symptom for you?
- YES ↓
- NO ↓

Is your poo often loose and frequent?
- NO ↓
- YES ↓

Are you constipated or do you often have hard poos?
- NO → Is your poo often loose and frequent?
- YES ↓

Do you often skip meals or eat a lot of processed foods?
- NO ↓
- YES ↓

Have you ever had an extreme reaction to food such as vomiting and diarrhoea or a rash?
- YES ↓

Does your tummy flare up when you're stressed?
- YES ↓
- NO ↓

Do you ever get a funny taste in your mouth, burning in your throat, or pain in your torso?
- NO →
- YES ↓

IT COULD BE... A food intolerance or allergy

IT COULD BE... Irritable Bowel Syndrome (IBS)

IT COULD BE... Lack of fibre/good nutrition

IT COULD BE... Indigestion

• SCIENCE •

What do your results mean...

FOOD INTOLERANCE OR ALLERGY

For some people, certain foods can lead to food-hypersensitivity. 'These reactions either involve the immune system, which is a "food allergy" or in cases where it doesn't, it's called a "food intolerance",' explains Dr Emma Williams, Waitrose Nutrition Manager.
SORT IT
Food allergy: Immediate reactions usually take place within two hours of eating, with the development of classic allergy symptoms such as, an itchy rash, swelling and in some cases, vomiting

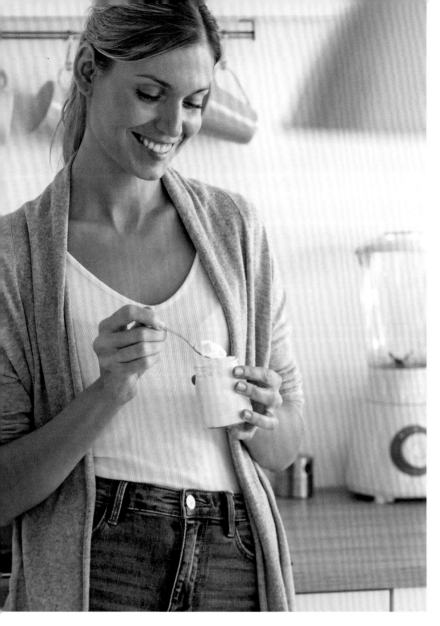

diagnosis to rule out other conditions such as coeliac or inflammatory bowel disease, so speak to your GP.

Bloating and wind: 'Avoid gas-producing foods such as beans, pulses, Brussels sprouts, sugar-free mints or gum and include oats and linseeds in your diet,' says Dr Williams.

Diarrhoea: 'Avoid sugar-free sweets or mints, or drinks containing sweeteners such as xylitol, sorbitol and mannitol. Limit caffeinated drinks to no more than three per day and reduce your intake of high-fibre foods. Stay hydrated.

LACK OF FIBRE/ GOOD NUTRITION

The average adult only consumes 18g of fibre per day – 12g lower than the recommended 30g intake. Fibre removes waste and toxins from the body and helps the digestive tract function. It also helps keep cholesterol low and stabilise blood-sugar levels, reducing type 2 diabetes risk.

SORT IT

'Adding more daily fibre should soften stools, helping them to pass out easier,' says Dr Williams. 'But avoid eating extra wheat bran as this can make constipation worse.' Fibre-rich foods include wholegrains, berries, oranges, nuts, seeds and broccoli and are packed with iron, and vitamins B and C.'

INDIGESTION

It's caused by stomach acid irritating the stomach lining or throat, giving a burning sensation or a full, bloated feeling. While unpleasant, it doesn't require medical assistance unless the symptoms continue past three weeks, or you have other difficulties.

SORT IT

'Limit caffeinated or alcoholic drinks and don't eat three to four hours before bed, avoiding any rich, spicy or fatty foods,' says Dr Williams. If stomach acid prevents you sleeping, prop up your head and shoulders in bed to stop the acid rising. Certain medications, such as ibuprofen or aspirin, may also make indigestion worse.

and diarrhoea. 'These can lead to serious problems, so seek urgent medical advice,' says Dr Williams.

Food intolerance: Symptoms such as bloating or tummy pain often come on several hours after eating. Keeping a food diary will help you to identify possible triggers. Try eliminating certain foods for two to six weeks to see whether things improve.

IRRITABLE BOWEL SYNDROME (IBS)

'Symptoms vary from person to person but typical signs include tummy discomfort, bloating, or a change in bowel movements for at least six months – often made worse by eating,' says Dr Williams. Passing mucus, feeling lethargic, experiencing nausea, bladder issues and backache are also indicators IBS can be brought on by stress.

SORT IT

It's important to have a confirmed

Diet

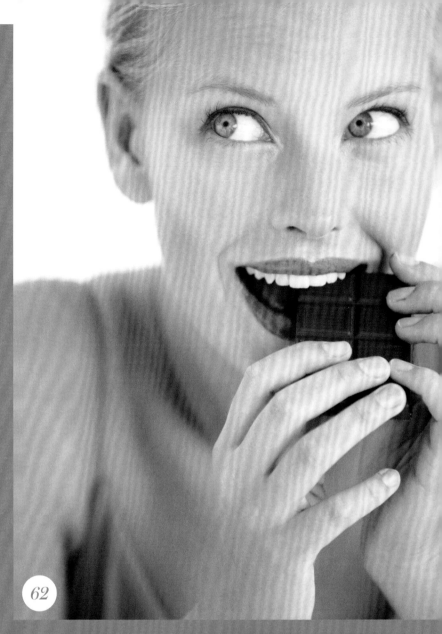

62

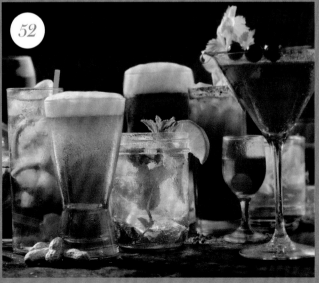

52

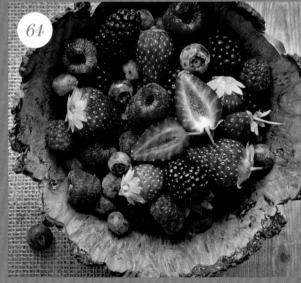

64

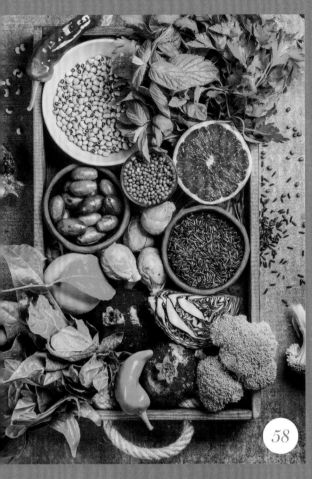

58

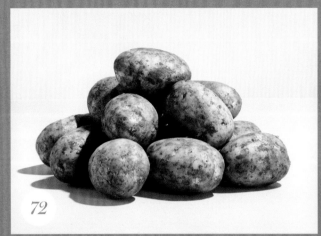

72

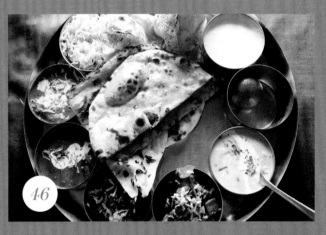

46

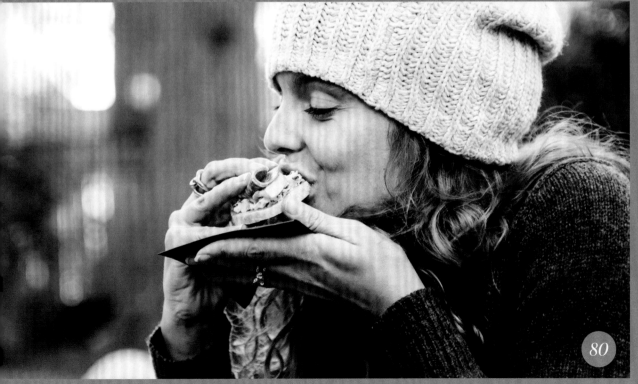

80

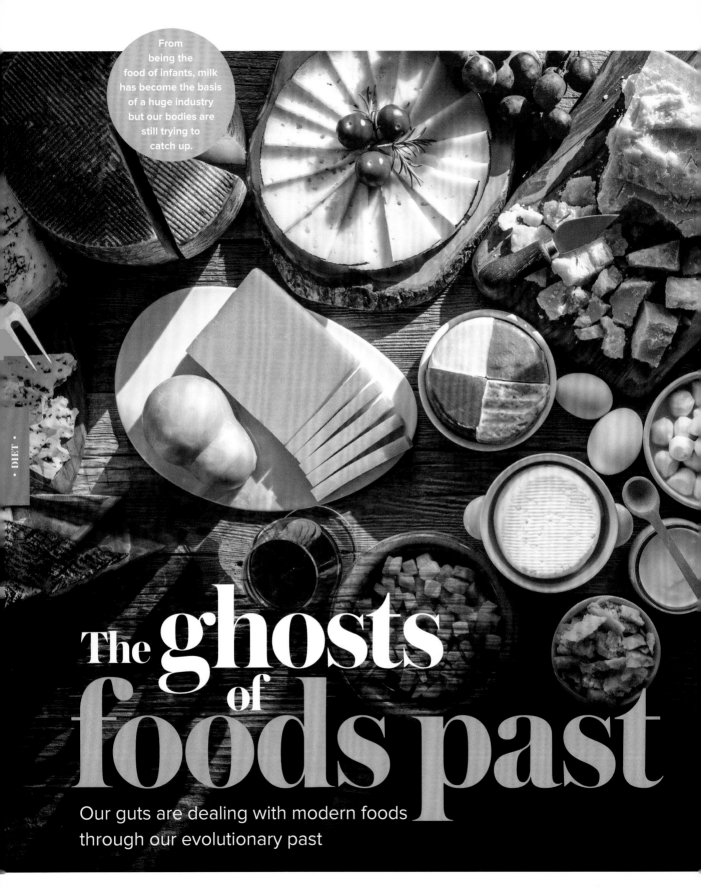

From being the food of infants, milk has become the basis of a huge industry but our bodies are still trying to catch up.

The ghosts of foods past

Our guts are dealing with modern foods through our evolutionary past

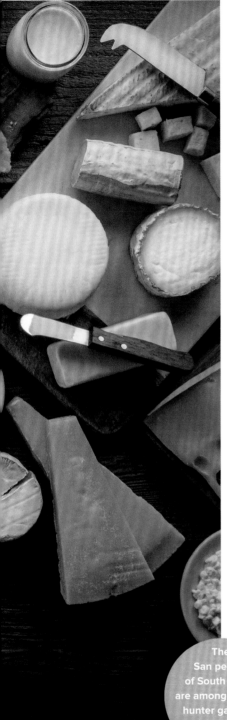

Human beings, Homo sapiens, first appeared on earth about **300,000** years ago. We were a wondering and a wandering species that migrated out from Africa, gradually colonising every part of the world.

For 287,000 of those 300,000 years, we were nomadic hunter gatherers, following the tracks of herds of game and visiting favoured sites to pick seasonal fruits or to trap migrating fish and animals. It was only with the invention of agriculture around 9,000 BCE that it became possible for people to settle down in one place.

The settling down also produced a growing population, which went on to create more complex social units and, to regulate and record all this, writing. The whole of recorded human history stretches back just 6,000 years, that is a mere two per cent of the total time human beings have been alive.

OUR NOMADIC PAST TODAY

Given that we spent so long as nomads, it's not surprising that our past still haunts our present, even though the lives we live today are so different from those of our ancestors. We see that in how difficult our bodies find sitting down all day because our bodies were made for walking. And we feel it with what we eat. Studies on the few remaining hunter gatherer peoples that maintain their

'Farmers naturally concentrate on the plants that produce the best crops and improving them'

ancient lifestyle indicate that they ate a huge variety of foodstuffs during the course of the year – food was, of course, seasonal. A nomad family would eat up to 500 different plants, roots, herbs and fruit during a normal year, with nearly as much variety in the animal food they consumed. By comparison, while today we have much more food to eat, the variety has greatly reduced to only 17 main plant crops. We use these plants in a huge number of different ways, but the absolute number of plants we eat has gone down dramatically. This is because farmers naturally concentrate on the plants that produce the best crops and improving them, rather than trying out low-yield plants.

The other huge change in our diets is milk and dairy products. Before the domestication of goats and cattle, the only milk we drank came from our mother's breast milk. To digest lactose,

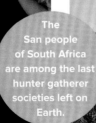

The San people of South Africa are among the last hunter gatherer societies left on Earth.

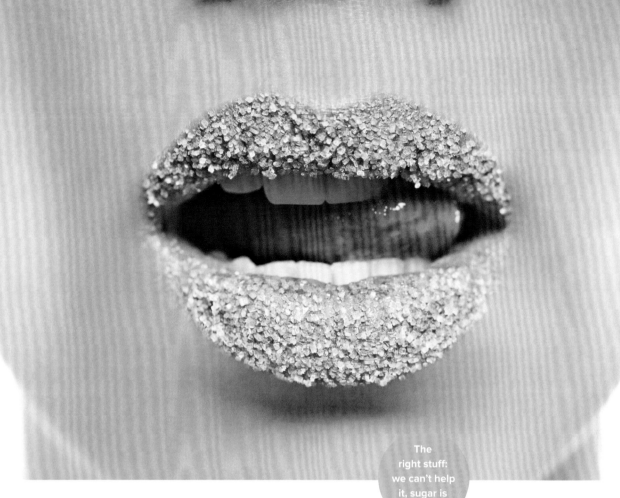

our small intestine excretes an enzyme during infancy, but our bodies were set to stop excreting this enzyme as we got older – after all, there was not much point in continuing to produce this enzyme when we stopped drinking milk that our mothers provided us with as they breastfed us.

But while we now continue eating and drinking dairy products into our old age, our bodies are only just beginning to catch up. 25 per cent of people now continue to produce the lactose-consuming enzyme in undiminished quantities throughout their lives. But for three-quarters of the world's population, the production of the lactose-consuming enzyme slows down as they age.

Luckily, lactose intolerance does not produce too much in the way of ill effects. Undigested dairy products provide a bonanza for the gut flora in the large intestine, leading to the production of gas. But a good camembert is probably worth a

fart or two, although stomach bloating and diarrhoea might suggest cutting back on the cheese.

DOES WHAT WE EAT MATTER?

This might seem like a strange question in these diet-conscious times, but it's an important question nonetheless.

The right stuff: we can't help it, sugar is sweet.

Everything we eat is broken down by the actions of the gut into sugars, amino acids and fats. On the basic chemical level, it makes no difference if we eat a bowl of quinoa and tofu or a Big Mac and fries. When the food gets to the small intestine, it's all become one of those three. So if everything is broken down to the same

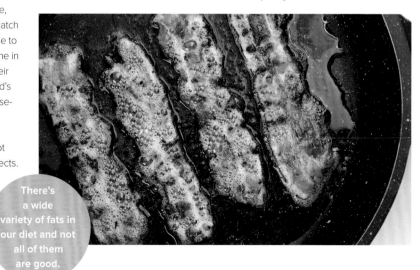

There's a wide variety of fats in our diet and not all of them are good.

> *'On the basic chemical level, it makes no difference if we eat a bowl of quinoa and tofu or a Big Mac'*

three classes of substances, why should it matter what we consume in the first place?

The problem lies in the change in what we eat. In particular, the discovery of how to grow and process sugar. While sugar cane was grown in India from prehistory, it was a rare and difficult crop, and expensive. Honey was the only sweetener available to the vast majority of mankind.

Sugar only began to spread when the secret of crystallising it was discovered in the 5th century CE during the Gupta Empire. Sugar crystals were called khanda, from which the word candy comes. Sugar production exploded following the European settlement of the New World, with vast plantations in the West Indies producing sugar cane as part of the Triangular Trade that took slaves from Africa, traded them for sugar and sugar derived products in the West Indies and then sailed back to Europe to buy goods to take south to Africa to trade with African slave dealers for the next round of slaves.

The problem with sugar is that the body loves it. Most people have a sweet tooth. It's a flavour that carries only positive connotations. That was all fine when the only sweet things we would normally eat were fruit and honey. But today, much processed food has sugar added. It's worth distinguishing between mechanically processed food, such as pasteurised milk and sausages, and chemically processed foods, such as breakfast cereals and ready meals. The latter usually have sugar added. Even

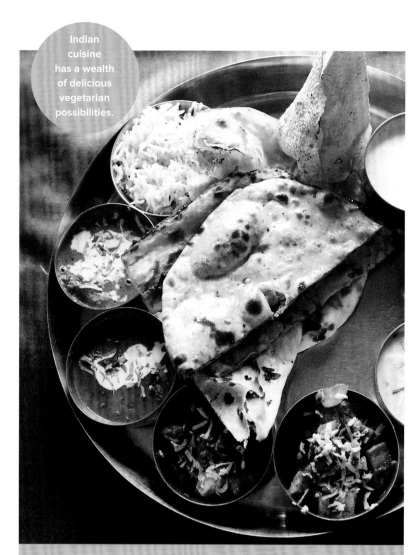

Indian cuisine has a wealth of delicious vegetarian possibilities.

GETTING YOUR PROTEIN FIX

Where to get the building blocks for the body

Proteins consist of chains of amino acids. There are 20 amino acids and they can be linked into an almost infinite variety of chains. Our DNA, the information template for the cells in our body, makes use of this density to instruct the development and maintenance of our bodies. The gut breaks down proteins into their constituent amino acids, which can then be absorbed directly through the gut wall and used in building proteins in our bodies. The richest source of proteins are other animals, for they contain the same building block proteins that we do. Most plants lack some of the key amino acids we need to maintain good health, so vegetarians and vegans need to supplement their diets with legumes and some of the few, but useful, plants that do contain the necessary proteins, such as quinoa. Tofu, made from soya milk, is another excellent source of protein, as are dairy products if those are a possibility. As two of the world's largest religions, Buddhism and Hinduism, prefer largely meat-free diets, there is a wealth of dietary experience to provide a healthy vegetarian existence for those who choose to forgo flesh in their food.

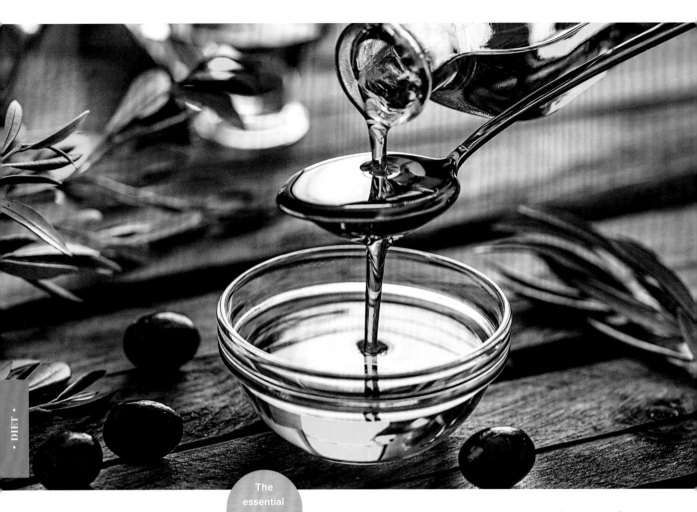

The essential good fat: olive oil.

without eating oven meals, we still have access to vastly more sweet foods and drinks than our ancestors. For our guts, still stuck in a pre-industrial world, all this sugar is a bonanza. Sugars require very little work on the part of our guts before they are absorbed.

Sugar is fuel. Imagine throwing petrol on a fire; it flares up in a blast of heat and flames, then dies down just as quickly. It's like that when we eat sugar. A surge of instant energy that sputters out. To cope with the inrush of sugar energy, the body also has to produce an equivalent rush of hormones, particularly insulin, to cope with the burst. The problem, of course, is that if we don't need this inrush of sugar energy, the body has to do something with it. The first step is to chain the sugars together again and make a substance called glycogen, which is stored in the

liver, and serves as a first-stop energy store. Rather annoyingly for people trying to lose weight, when we exercise, the body's first recourse is to its glycogen store. It's only after that is exhausted, which usually takes about an hour, that the body starts burning fat.

But sugar is not only sweet. Carbohydrates, the main constituents of bread, pasta, rice and indeed most of the things we eat, are actually strings of sugar molecules linked together. The key factor in determining what are the best carbohydrate foods to eat is how long it takes for the body to break the carbohydrates down into sugars. Eating white bread, for instance, is not much different, from the gut's point of view, to eating the same quantity of sugar. Wholegrain bread, on the other hand, contains more complex sugar chains that

take more work to break down. So the sugar rush is spread out, allowing the body to adjust more gradually.

FAT TIME

The life of a hunter gatherer often involved periods of dearth. Hunger stalked the hunting plains. In fact, the 21st century is the first time in history when there have been more fat people than starving people. Given so many generations where famine was the greater threat, our bodies have naturally evolved to eke every last bit of nourishment from the food we eat, and to store what we don't immediately need against future hunger. Unfortunately, the body can turn sugar into fat more easily than any other substance – even more easily than the fat we eat.

Fat is special. While for years it was the greasy cousin to bright, white Mr Sugar,

'As an energy store, fat holds twice the amount of energy per gram when compared to carbohydrates'

now we know that fat, at least in certain forms, is more beneficial than a spoonful of sugar, although it's hard to see fat becoming a refrain in a song as sugar has been so often. As an energy store, fat holds twice the amount of energy per gram when compared to carbohydrates and proteins. Fat sheathes our nerves, acting as an insulator, and coats every cell in our body as the main constituent of the cell membrane.

As well as making fat, the body absorbs it from our food. However, there's a problem: fat is insoluble. Where sugar can dissolve straight through the wall of the small intestine into the bloodstream, if fat did that, it would clog up the vessels leading to the liver (where the blood from the gut goes first, for a thorough check and clean).

Instead, it's the lymphatic system that absorbs fat. Lymph is the pale, straw-coloured fluid that you can see sometimes weeping from around wounds. Every capillary in the body has an accompanying lymph vessel, taking immune cells to where they are needed and draining excess fluid. The fat we eat is absorbed into the lymphatic system, joining the Ductus thoracicus, the biggest lymph vessel in the body. The lymph is a one-way system, driven by gravity, whose other main job is to drain the debris from cells and return it to the venous system, where the heart then circulates it back to the clean-up organs for removal from the body.

The drawback of this is that the fat we eat with our food and absorb via the gut is sent, via the venous system, directly to the heart without being cleaned up by the liver on the way. This means that the heart is exposed to whatever cheap fats the burger joint down the road bought in to fry their quarter pounders. Obviously, this is not great.

Good fats, such as cold-pressed (extra virgin) olive oil, can have considerable health benefits. Many studies have linked the consumption of good olive oil to reduced incidences of arteriosclerosis, Alzheimer's, chronic inflammation and macular degeneration. However, even good fats such as olive oil and other anti-inflammatory oils are only good in reasonable quantities.

The difficult fact is that we live in times when high-energy food is plentiful and cheap. The main food problem of the modern age is learning to live with having too much to eat. While it's definitely a better situation than trying to cope with not having enough to eat – the consequences of malnutrition are deeper, quicker and much more crippling than obesity – it nevertheless has its own set of challenges, which, because of our evolutionary history, may prove very difficult to solve.

It takes an hour of exercise before we start burning off fat.

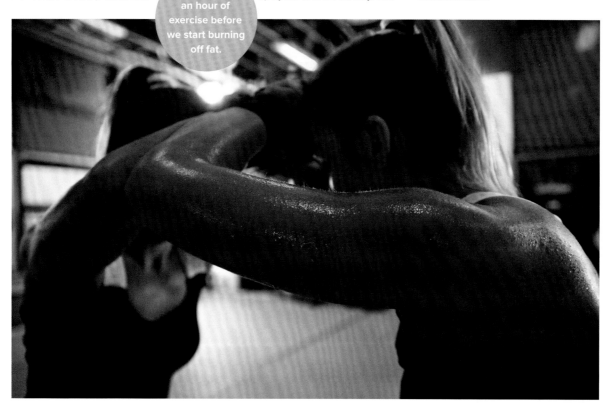

• DIET •

Worst foods
for your gut

Some of the best foods for our tastebuds are, in fact, the worst for our gut

t's no secret that many of the tastiest and most enjoyable things to eat and drink are bad for us. Those late-night cheesy chips play havoc with our waistlines, alcohol damages our livers and caffeine affects our sleep cycles. We all know that, but what is possibly less obvious is the impact certain foods and drinks have on our gut health.

Our digestive system is a fascinatingly delicate and diverse ecosystem of bacteria, all battling for supremacy. Your aim should be to populate your gut with good, healthy bacteria that helps everything to work as it should, but a poor diet could lead to an excess of bad bacteria, known as dysbiosis, and it doesn't end well for you. Too much bad bacteria, or not enough good, can result in bloating, gas, illness, disease, food intolerances and clogged arteries. Obviously you need a little bit of Epicurean joy in your life, but here are some of the things you should try and avoid an excess of if you want a happy, healthy gut.

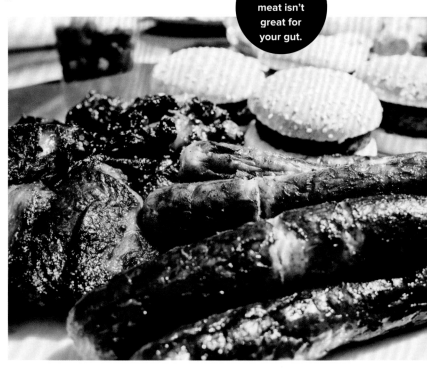

Red meat

A carnivorous diet could harm your gut

It's well known that red meat like beef, lamb and pork isn't great for you in large quantities as it can cause heart problems. However, it's less well known that this is partly due to its impact on your gut.

Animal cells contain molecules called carnitine. As humans are animals, we have carnitine in our bodies, so when we eat meat, this increases the amount of carnitine in our system. When digested, some of the carnitine reacts with our gut bacteria and creates another substance called trimethylamine N-oxide (TMAO). This has been linked to cardiovascular disease and a build-up of plaque in your arteries that is clearly very hazardous to your health. Our bodies are able to cope with a certain amount of extra carnitine so

you don't have to give up red meat entirely, but wolfing down a daily bacon butty or beefburger could prove too much for it to handle.

Studies have shown that switching between a meat- and a plant-based diet can have an effect on your body in as little as 24 hours, so a couple of days per week where you switch meat for a plant-based alternative, such as tofu, can help your body process the carnitine in your gut without too many adverse effects.

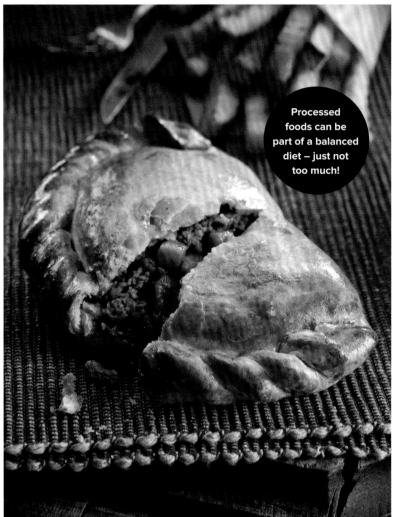

Processed foods can be part of a balanced diet – just not too much!

Artificial sweeteners

Fake sugar isn't so sweet for your gut

You may think that using artificial sweetener in your tea or coffee (more on that later) instead of sugar is doing your body a favour as it doesn't have the same amount of calories. However, there are some hidden side effects to products like aspartame and saccharin. These sugar substitutes can actually transform good gut bacteria into bad pathogenic bacteria, which could cause serious illness if they cross into the bloodstream. This includes sepsis, organ failure and glucose intolerance. As the aim is to have as much good bacteria and as little bad in our guts as possible, an excess of artificial sweetener is the absolute enemy of good gut health and should be avoided where possible. A little bit of natural sugar, honey or good old fruit juice can go a long way in adding a bit of sweetness into your body in more ways than one.

Processed foods

These foods are tough to process

Processed foods, such as cheese, bacon and pasties, aren't great for your general health, and can also cause issues for your gut. They are generally foodstuffs that have been heavily modified and altered as well as being loaded with sugar and salt to make them taste nice.

As a result, a lot of the goodness in the base ingredients is lost during processing. That means that not only are you not getting much fibre or good bacteria, but by filling up on processed food, you aren't eating the kinds of foods that your gut really needs.

About 75 per cent of the world's food supply comes from just 12 plants and five animals, something that negatively affects our gut's bacteria diversity levels, and people in Europe and North America have less diverse gut flora than those in rural Africa and South America. Much of this is put down to a Western diet that is made up of too much processed food and not enough natural produce.

As with everything, a balance is important here. It's not the end of the world to have some processed foods in your diet, but you need to make sure you're making up for them by having plenty of food that's extra-good for your gut health.

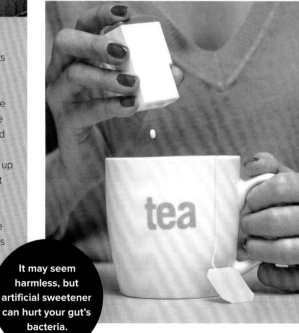

It may seem harmless, but artificial sweetener can hurt your gut's bacteria.

Antibiotics

Good for your health, bad for your gut

Antibiotics help humans get over all kinds of illnesses and diseases, but they're also used on animals, making their way into the food chain. They work by killing bacteria, but they aren't able to determine the difference between good and bad. Therefore, if you eat meat that still contains traces of antibiotics, you could be killing off both good and bad bacteria in your gut, reducing the quantity of gut flora.

Our guts have an internal clock that regulates the bacteria levels. If it is thrown off, it can lead to Type 2 diabetes and weight gain. This isn't necessarily a short-term issue either, and it can take a long time for your body to restore your gut's bacteria levels to what they were before, so be careful with your meat.

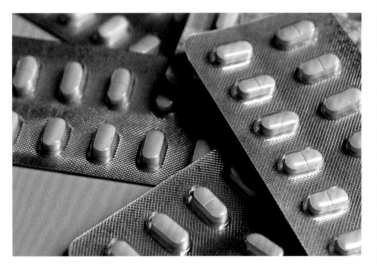

Deep fried food is harder to digest.

Fried food

The fast way to bad gut health

Fast, fried food such as chips, burgers and battered fish is bad for your gut as well as your waistline. When food is deep fried in copious amounts of oil, it makes it much harder for your body to digest.

Have you ever feasted on a meal of fried chicken and chips and felt uncomfortably full for much longer than when having eaten a similarly sized meal? That's because your digestive system is having to work harder to break the food down and that can lead to all kinds of stomach trouble, such as flatulence and diarrhoea. Also, some experts believe that the chemical changes in oil that has been heated can hurt the good bacteria in your gut and cause bad bacteria to multiply. Some oil is fine, but your gut won't thank you if you bombard it with loads of the stuff.

Alcohol **Drinking can make your gut whine**

Red wine in small quantities is actually good for the diversity of your gut's diversity, but drinking to excess can have the reverse effect. Too much boozing can change your gut's microbiome negatively, causing the amount of bad bacteria to outweigh the good, which is even worse than a full Sunday hangover.

Your head won't thank you for overdoing the booze – and neither will your gut.

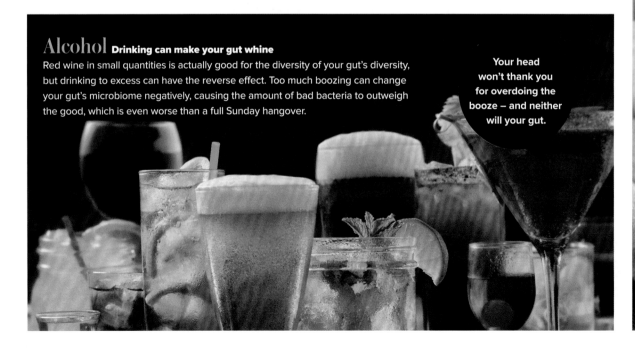

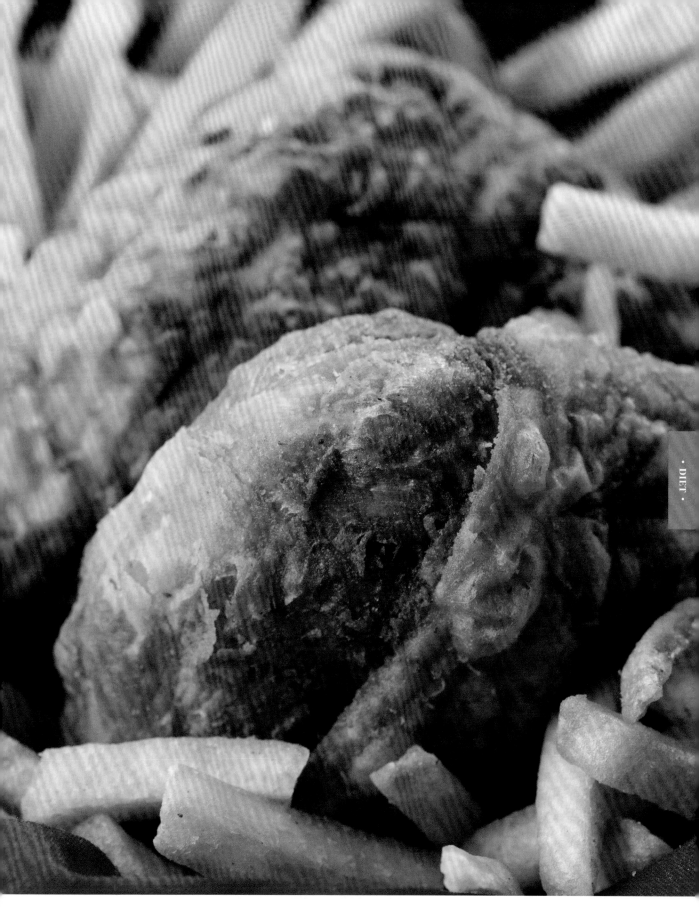

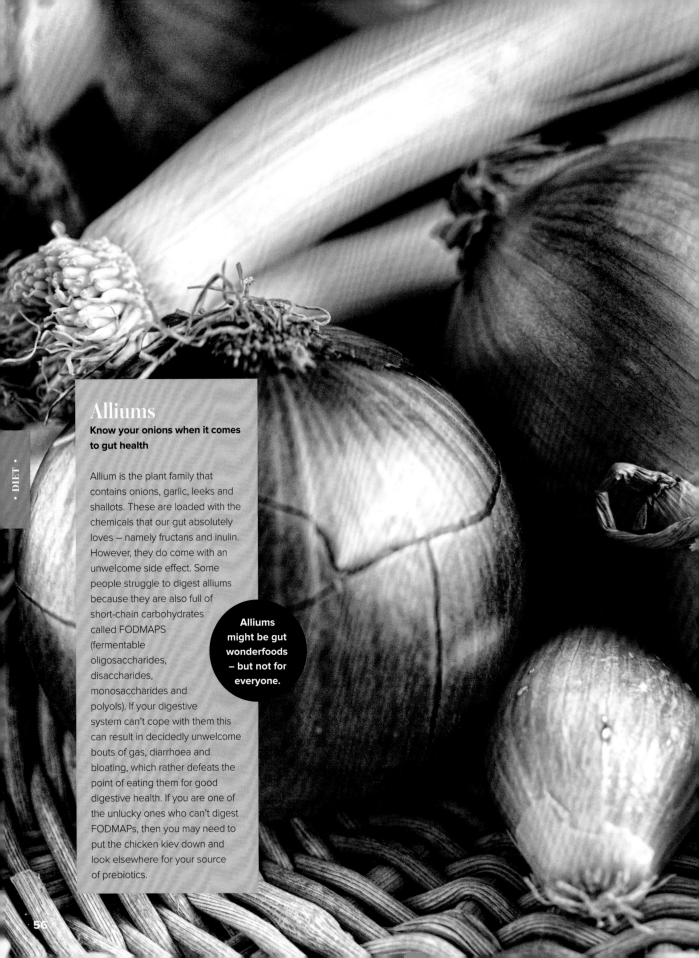

Alliums

Know your onions when it comes to gut health

Allium is the plant family that contains onions, garlic, leeks and shallots. These are loaded with the chemicals that our gut absolutely loves — namely fructans and inulin. However, they do come with an unwelcome side effect. Some people struggle to digest alliums because they are also full of short-chain carbohydrates called FODMAPS (fermentable oligosaccharides, disaccharides, monosaccharides and polyols). If your digestive system can't cope with them this can result in decidedly unwelcome bouts of gas, diarrhoea and bloating, which rather defeats the point of eating them for good digestive health. If you are one of the unlucky ones who can't digest FODMAPs, then you may need to put the chicken kiev down and look elsewhere for your source of prebiotics.

Alliums might be gut wonderfoods — but not for everyone.

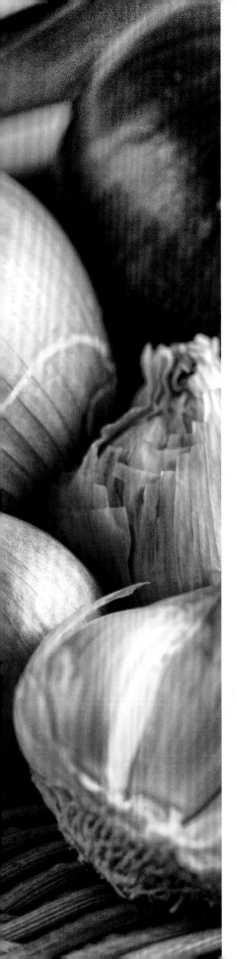

Dairy

Certain dairy can be scary for your gut

Yoghurt, especially yoghurt that contains live cultures, is one of the products that is the best for populating your gut with healthy, good bacteria. However, not all dairy is equal. Unfermented dairy, such as milk and cheese, can have a negative effect on the bacteria within your gut, changing it quite dramatically and putting you at risk of intestinal illness. Limiting your dairy intake can help to keep your gut in a normal, balanced state.

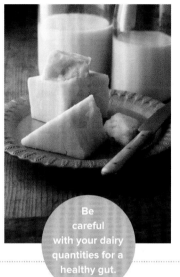

Be careful with your dairy quantities for a healthy gut.

Caffeine might help us stay awake, but it wreaks havoc in the gut.

Caffeine

Your morning pick-me-up may be getting you down

Most of us love a coffee or a tea first thing in the morning, and there aren't many of us who haven't reached for a Red Bull when falling asleep at our desks. There are polyphenols in caffeine that are good for the gut, but be warned, too much caffeine also has a highly stimulating effect on our stomachs. When caffeine passes through your intestines, it makes the process of food moving through your gut speed up, thus making you need to go and sit on the toilet fairly urgently. This isn't disastrous, but it isn't ideal to force food through your digestive system faster than it wants to, so try and limit your caffeine intake where possible.

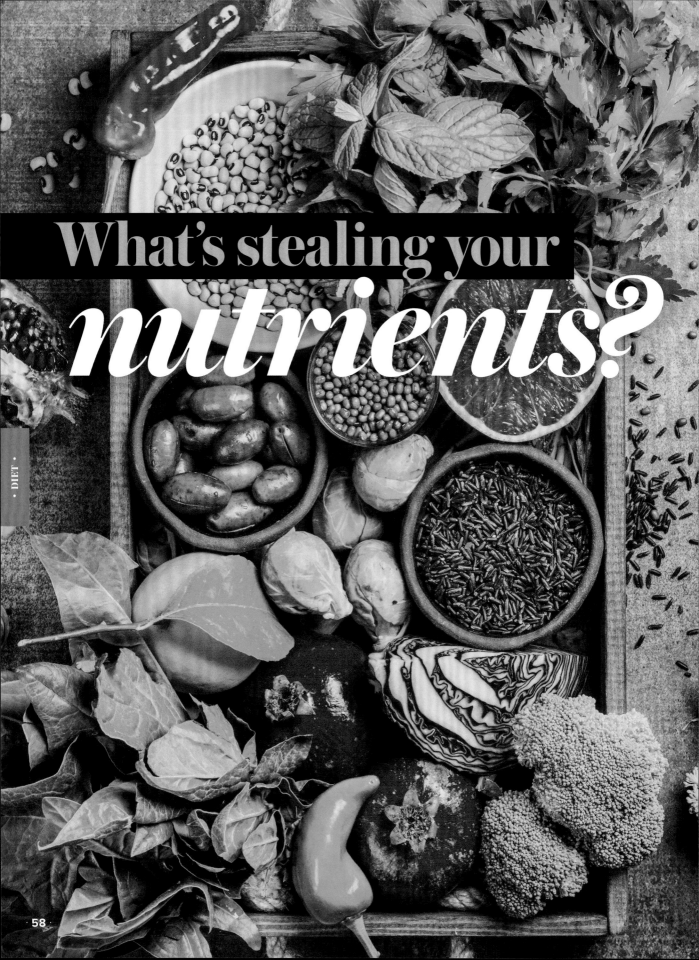

What's stealing your *nutrients?*

You eat right, take supplements, sleep well so why do you feel so exhausted? These habits could be sapping your body of nutrients...

Do you often feel tired, even though you eat well, exercise and get enough sleep? Or, perhaps, you suffer from achy muscles and low mood? If there are no medical causes, it could be down to lifestyle choices.

'We need sufficient nutrients to stay healthy and, ideally, we'd get what we need from our diets,' says registered nutritionist Rob Hobson. 'But, sometimes, no matter how healthy you try to be, some of the things you do every day may be unwittingly hijacking your ability to obtain the nutrients you need.'

'Many people are not aware that certain lifestyle factors may be sabotaging their nutrient intake,' adds Mike Wakeman, clinical pharmacist, specialising in nutritional medicine. 'Research shows, for example, that 84 per cent of the top 20 most commonly used medications affect nutrient status. As multiple medication use is common in the UK, the accumulative effect is causing massive nutrient deficiencies.'

From an evening aperitif, to demanding workloads, a multitude of everyday issues could be to blame.

The nutrient thieves

TEA AND COFFEE

Do you like to finish a meal with a tea or coffee? You may be depleting your iron stores. 'Tannins found in tea, and chlorogenic acid found in coffee, are natural compounds that can reduce iron absorption,' says Rob. 'Research shows having tea with a meal may inhibit iron uptake by around 60 per cent and drinking coffee within an hour of a meal can reduce iron absorption by 80 per cent. Tea and coffee also reduce absorption of other minerals such as magnesium, calcium and zinc.'

WHAT TO DO

'Wait at least one hour after eating before you have a cup of tea or coffee,' says Rob. 'Take supplements with water, as a hot drink will stop the nutrients being absorbed. Take iron supplements with orange juice, as vitamin C aids absorption, or choose a liquid supplement that is gentler on the stomach.'

OVER-EXERCISING

'Strenuous exercise can cause you to become depleted in antioxidant vitamins A, C, E, B, iron, and electrolyte salts and minerals, including sodium, potassium, magnesium and calcium,' says Rob. 'Deficiencies can leave you continuously tired and make it harder to recover after a workout. Symptoms of low magnesium – vital for energy – include weakness and muscle cramps. If you're pale, breathless and weak, you may be low in iron, or even anaemic, especially if you have heavy periods.'

WHAT TO DO

'Make sure you're eating enough to meet your energy requirements for exercise, including protein, which you need for healthy muscles,' says Rob. Foods high in iron include lentils, liver, shellfish, pumpkin seeds, quinoa and tofu. For magnesium eat dark leafy greens, nuts and seeds, and oily fish. 'Get your calcium from almonds, broccoli and dairy. All veg, avocado and bananas contain potassium,' says Rob. 'Take a multivitamin and mineral every day.'

ALCOHOL

'Alcohol can deplete you of vitamins B and C, and minerals, potassium, magnesium and zinc,' explains Rob. 'Your body needs B vitamins to enable enzymes to metabolise alcohol in the liver. So, the more you drink, the quicker you'll use up B vitamins, which are crucial for energy, brain health and the nervous system. Alcohol also has a diuretic effect, which means vitamins B and C (which are water soluble), potassium, magnesium and zinc are more easily flushed out of the system. Alcohol also reduces digestive enzymes, which means the absorption of nutrients is inhibited.'

WHAT TO DO

'If you're having a drink, line your stomach – something like a tuna mayonnaise sandwich, which has protein, fat and carbohydrate. This will slow the rate alcohol enters your bloodstream,' says Rob. 'Eat more fruit and vegetables that contain vitamin C, and foods high in vitamin B (such as brown rice, eggs and lentils.' You could also take daily vitamin B and C supplements to top up and ensure there's enough in your system to keep you healthy.

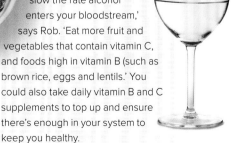

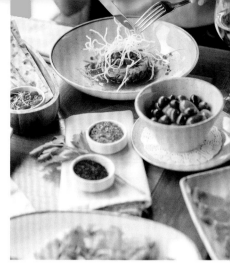

SUNSCREEN

'If you spend a lot of time indoors, covered up, or you wear sunscreen every day this lowers the amount of vitamin D you absorb from sunlight. Figures show that one in five people are deficient in vitamin D in the UK, and in winter around 40 per cent are,' reveals Rob who explains we need vitamin D to absorb calcium, and phosphate from our diet and to keep our bones, teeth, muscles and immune system healthy. He adds, 'Research also suggests if you're low in vitamin D, you're more susceptible to flu and colds, heart disease, cancer and diabetes.'

WHAT TO DO

'Spend at least 20 minutes in sunlight every day. If you have darker skin you may need longer,' says Rob. 'Leave face, forearms, hands and/or lower legs uncovered, without sunscreen. But add sunscreen if you plan to be out longer. You can also eat more foods that contain vitamin D (oily fish, eggs, mushrooms) and take a supplement – 10mcg (400 iu) daily.'

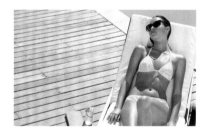

THE PILL

'A number of studies, including a report by the World Health Organization (WHO), have identified oral contraceptives as having an impact upon nutritional status,' says Mike. 'The research shows that oral contraceptives can lower a woman's level of folic acid, vitamins A, B1, B2, B6, B12, C and E, as well as magnesium, zinc, selenium, copper, co-enzyme Q10 and beta carotene.' He adds that there are also concerns the pill may reduce the absorption of folic acid, a deficiency of which may lead to foetal abnormalities, if pregnancy occurs while taking the pill, or shortly after taking it.

WHAT TO DO

'As well as eating a highly nutritious diet, take a multivitamin and mineral supplement. Also, a folic acid supplement, especially if you're planning on trying to conceive in the near future.' Mike also recommends seeing a nutritional therapist, or your GP, to check for any nutritional deficiencies if you are concerned.

ASPIRIN

'Taking the occasional aspirin, for a headache, is fine,' says Dr Sarah Brewer, GP and medical nutritionist. 'But, if you take it regularly, even in small doses, it can increase the risk of ulcers and bleeding. This is because aspirin blocks the absorption of vitamin C, which has a protective effect on the stomach lining.'

WHAT TO DO

Dr Brewer adds, 'If you're taking aspirin long term (eg, to reduce the risk of heart attack), take a daily vitamin C supplement. Ensure you also get vitamin C from your diet by eating plenty of fresh fruit and vegetables.'

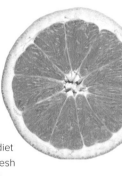

STRESS

'When you're stressed, your body uses vitamins B and C, and the mineral magnesium more quickly,' says Rob. 'Yet, these are exactly the nutrients you need to help your body cope with stress. B vitamins are crucial to keep your nervous system healthy; they support brain function, regulate mood and are involved in energy production.' As for vitamin C, it helps to support the adrenal glands, and magnesium, known as "nature's tranquilliser", also plays an important role in supporting the body when you're stressed. Magnesium helps to regulate heart rate, lowers blood pressure and stimulates levels of the calming neurotransmitter, GABA (gamma-aminobutyric acid) in the brain.'

WHAT TO DO

'Make sure each mouthful you eat is highly nutritious, especially if you are under more pressure than normal,' says Rob. 'Foods high in B vitamins include wholegrains, sunflower seeds, almonds, avocados and sweet potatoes. Vitamin C is found in citrus fruits, kiwi, strawberries and vegetables.' As well as the magnesium-rich foods listed, include kidney beans, chickpeas, salmon, mackerel, tuna and dark chocolate (over 70 per cent cacao). Rob adds: 'To reduce stress try meditation, yoga or mindfulness and think about other lifestyle changes you can make.'

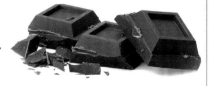

• DIET •

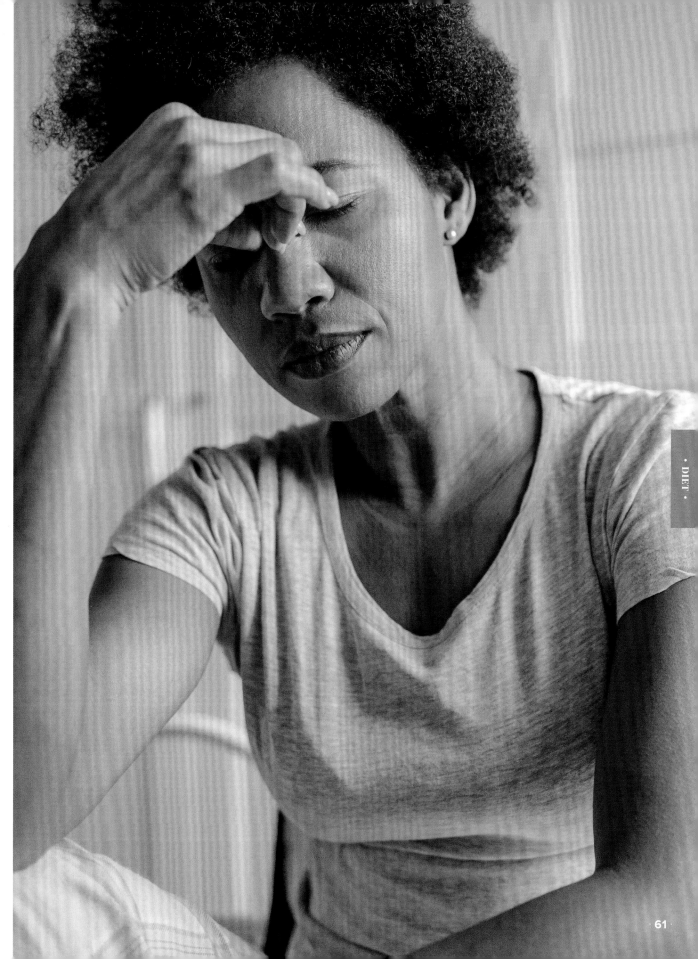

Decode that CRAVING

Desperate for chocolate? Eager for a packet of crisps? A recurring yearning for salty snacks or something sweet after a meal could indicate an underlying issue. We asked the experts...

Do you control your cravings, or do they control you? If it's the latter, your body might be trying to tell you you're missing something. 'Cravings can be put down to greed, but they are more likely to be a biochemical urge that is almost impossible to control by mind power alone,' says nutritionist Dr Marilyn Glenville. 'Your body is demanding a particular type of food because it has a need for it, and it will let you know in no uncertain terms.' Hence why we can't move on from the afternoon slump without chocolate. Here, the experts reveal what your cravings might really mean.

You're desperate for stodgy carbs

Whether it's doughy bread or a big bowl of pasta, Dr Glenville explains that 'carb cravings are a sign of low levels of tryptophan, needed for serotonin production – a "happy" brain chemical.' She adds: 'It plays a crucial role in sleep and wake cycles, as well as digestion and a lack of it can lead to low mood and anxiety.' And if you're after something carby and sugary (such as a doughnut or cake), you might have low dopamine levels too. 'The combination of fat and sugar can

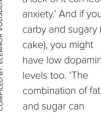

have quite a unique effect on your brain,' says nutritionist Emma Ross. 'There's some evidence to suggest that when fat is added to the equation, it can trigger the release of dopamine – a neurotransmitter that is associated with pleasure and reward.'

CURB THE CRAVING
✛ Stock up on turkey, eggs, bananas and walnuts, which all contain tryptophan. 'Try including omega-3 rich oily fish or flaxseeds in your diet and giving your dopamine levels a boost. Taking more exercise can also trigger dopamine pathways,' says Emma.

You've just got to have chocolate

Can't get through the day without it? 'Chocolate cravings can be a sign of a magnesium deficiency,' explains Emma. 'In the lead-up to a period – or during the menopause – you're more at risk of being deficient in magnesium,' she says. What's more, magnesium plays a part in bone health, preventing inflammation, maintaining a steady healthy blood pressure, easing anxiety and balancing the nervous system.

CURB THE CRAVING
✛ Rather than turning to chocolate, opt for more wholegrains, beans, nuts and green leafy vegetables in your diet to help top up your magnesium. However, if you're in real need of a chocolate fix, eat a piece of dark chocolate (but make sure it's at least 70 per cent cocoa solids). The added benefit of swapping milk chocolate for dark chocolate is that it's richer and harder to overindulge.

You've a thirst for something fizzy

You might be dehydrated. 'The combination of a fizzy sensation with a sweet taste can be pleasurable and stimulating, and it can seem to quench your thirst better than non-carbonated drinks,' says nutritionist Cassandra Barns.

CURB THE CRAVING
✛ Choose sparkling water to quench your thirst and then gradually adjust to still water. If you find water boring, try infusing it with citrus, cucumber or berries. Aim to drink 2 litres of water per day.

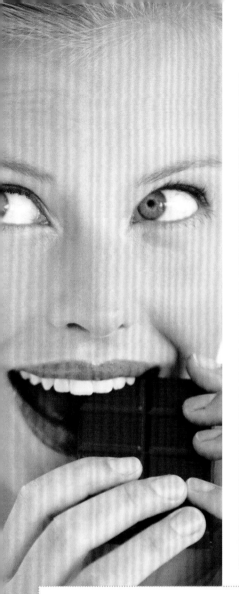

You've got a hankering for a hot curry

If you're wanting a warming curry, it could be your body's way of telling you that your immune system needs a boost. Spicy food is renowned for its antioxidant-rich spices, making chilli, turmeric and ginger perfect for combating a cold. Capsaicin, the substance that gives chillies their fiery kick, also stimulates the release of endorphins. Craving spice may also be a sign of a zinc deficiency, which regulates our taste and smell. If levels are too low, we struggle to taste blander foods.

CURB THE CRAVING

✛ **'Eat a curry – but make your own with good-quality meat, such as organic chicken, or go veggie with butternut squash and chickpeas,' says Cassandra. 'Use a little bit of coconut oil, and go for tomato-based sauces rather than creamy.' To up your zinc intake, eat eggs, fish and pumpkin seeds and support your immune system with plenty of vitamin C by eating oranges and leafy veg.**

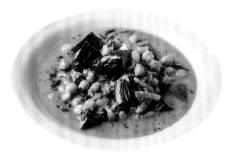

You're seeking something salty

If you feel like diving into a packet of crisps, you may be low on sodium. 'If you crave salty food, it could mean your sodium levels have fallen too low, usually due to dehydration after exercise, illness or drinking alcohol,' says nutritionist Shona Wilkinson. 'Sodium is an important mineral that helps maintain water balance in our body and also regulates blood pressure.' Craving salty foods is also a symptom of adrenal exhaustion, meaning your body needs the additional minerals found in natural salt. Zinc is the main mineral used in the body's reaction to stress and can disrupt the salt balance in the body. It also affects your sense of taste, resulting in a penchant for salty flavours.

CURB THE CRAVING

✛ **Try to minimise your stress where possible and, because salt is addictive, retrain your taste buds by swapping salt for seaweed granules. The sodium content is just 3.5 per cent compared with around 40 per cent in regular salt. If your craving persists, try a handful of nuts, seeds, olives, a small portion of salted popcorn, dried anchovies or fresh celery sticks and carrots.**

• DIET •

You REALLY need biscuits

Sugar is addictive and we soon crave our next fix if we go too long without it. You could also crave sugar when you get an energy slump because your blood sugar levels have dropped too low. Tiredness can make us reach for sugary snacks, as a lack of sleep leads to an increase of ghrelin, the hormone that triggers appetite. What's more, a chromium deficiency can also affect your blood glucose levels.

CURB THE CRAVING

✛ **The worst thing you can do is succumb to refined sources of sugar, as they give a short-lived boost of energy, followed by a sharp dip, leaving energy levels even** lower than before. **'For a sweet taste, try figs or passion fruit, which also contain soluble fibre that will help to slow the release of sugar into your bloodstream and avoid any extreme fluctuations,' explains Emma. Opt for low glycaemic (low GI) foods that provide sustained energy, such as crudités or oatcakes with houmous, or a handful of walnuts, and eat regular meals to balance your blood sugar. A chromium supplement, or adding cinnamon to your meals, can also help deter you from the biscuit jar.**

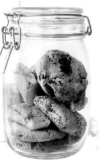

Best foods
for a
healthy gut

Find out how to feed your way
to a gut bursting with good bacteria

Food plays a huge part in regulating the health of your gut. Just like a car requires the right kind of fuel, oil and care to keep all its parts running smoothly, your body needs the right kinds of foods in the right quantities to keep everything working.

There are about 100 trillion bacteria in your gut, some good and some bad. Keeping the good bacteria high in both quantity and quality is vital to keeping you healthy. A gut full of good bacteria can aid digestion, fight disease, reduce stress, increase energy levels and maintain healthy weight, skin and hair.

The key things to look out for in gut-friendly foods are probiotics, prebiotics, polyphenols and fibre. At their most basic, probiotics help create good bacteria, prebiotics help feed them, polyphenols attack bad bacteria and fibre keeps things moving. Most natural foods contain at least one of these, but not all are created equal.

Sauerkraut

There's nothing sour about this probiotic-rich food

Probiotics are one of the most crucial parts of a good gut diet and what starts the whole process off. These are live bacteria that are created when foods such as sauerkraut, kimchi, miso and yoghurt go through the fermentation process. When the base product, whether it be dairy or cabbage, is broken down by microorganisms, it creates the acid that gives the above foods their slightly sour flavour. While this may not be to your personal taste, it creates the perfect environment for the probiotics to multiply, loading your meal with good bacteria.

When you then come to eat these probiotic-rich foods, this populates your gut with all the good bacteria it needs to help balance out the bad bacteria and achieve intestinal harmony. Yoghurt is probably the most readily available probiotic-full food available to Western shoppers (look out for the phrase "Live and Active cultures" on the carton because that is where the good stuff really is), but sauerkraut and kimchi are a step above.

Both are pickled cabbage, which gives you huge quantities of vitamin C, a key ally in the battle against disease while keeping your cells healthy. They're also a handy lactose-free alternative. As you'll see later on, an excess of dairy can lead to problems in the gut, whereas sauerkraut and kimchi provide just a whole lot of goodness for your stomach — if you are able to stomach the taste!

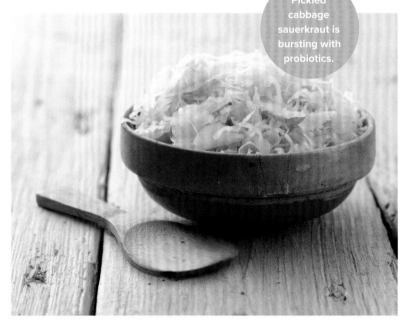

Pickled cabbage sauerkraut is bursting with probiotics.

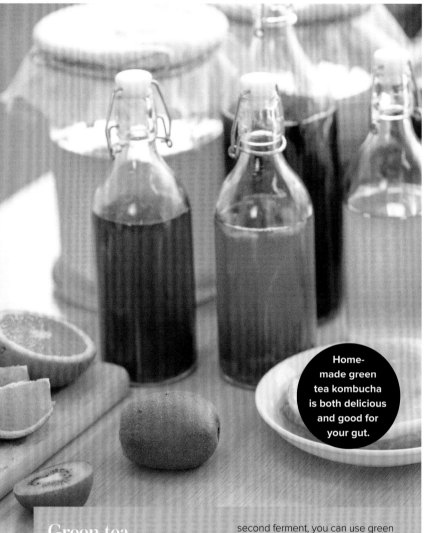

Home-made green tea kombucha is both delicious and good for your gut.

Chicory root
In for some inulin

Inulin is a type of fructan that is found in plant fibres and is also a good bacteria-feeding prebiotic. It helps your gut health through its ability to draw in water, making your faeces less firm and much easier to get rid of. Therefore foods high in inulin are great ways to avoid or relieve constipation.

Onion and garlic are both good, commonly eaten sources of inulin, but if you really want a major hit then try chicory root. This plant contains nearly 50g of inulin per 100g and is far and away the most concentrated natural form of the product, so much so that chicory root extract is what inulin supplements are made from.

You can boil chicory root and eat it as a side vegetable, or you can dry and roast it where it becomes a more than adequate coffee substitute.

Green tea kombucha
The drink that is pro-antioxidants

If you don't feel like eating all your probiotics, you can also drink them. The most easily picked-up liquid is a drink such as Yakult or Actimel but, just like yoghurt, they do contain dairy. Your best alternative is green tea kombucha.

This is a drink made by fermenting tea with sugar and a SCOBY (symbiotic culture of bacteria and yeast that you can create yourself or buy in a health shop) to create a fizzy, refreshing drink with just a hint of sourness. While it's commonly made with black tea and later flavoured with fruit during the second ferment, you can use green tea as the base, which is slightly lighter and fizzier.

Due to the fermentation process, kombucha is filled with probiotics that will help your gut boost its good bacteria numbers. Not only that, but choosing green tea over black means that your drink will also provide you with valuable antioxidants to help you fight disease, and contains less caffeine.

It is possible to brew your own kombucha at home or buy it in many high street health stores, but just be careful to watch out for added sweetener in store-bought kombucha, as this could cancel out any benefit of the drink.

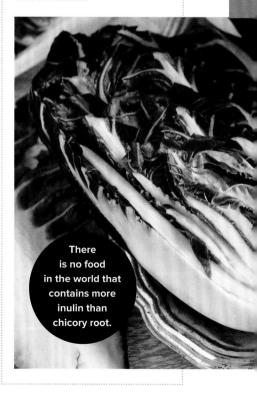

There is no food in the world that contains more inulin than chicory root.

Green bananas
Resistant starch is not futile

As well as inulin and fructans, resistant starch is a key element of building your healthy gut. This is a starch that can be found in foods such as green bananas, oats and nuts. It doesn't get digested in your stomach, so makes its way through to your colon where it feeds and fuels those good bacteria.

Most starchy food like potatoes and ripe bananas are digested early on in your digestive system, so these resistant starches are crucial to feeding that area further along your gut. As well as feeding those good bacteria, benefits of resistant starches include strengthening your colon's cells, reducing your risk of colon cancer and pumping short-chain fatty acids to your vital organs where they can do more good work.

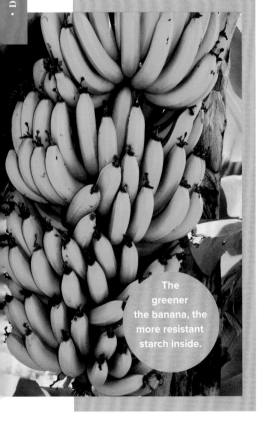

The greener the banana, the more resistant starch inside.

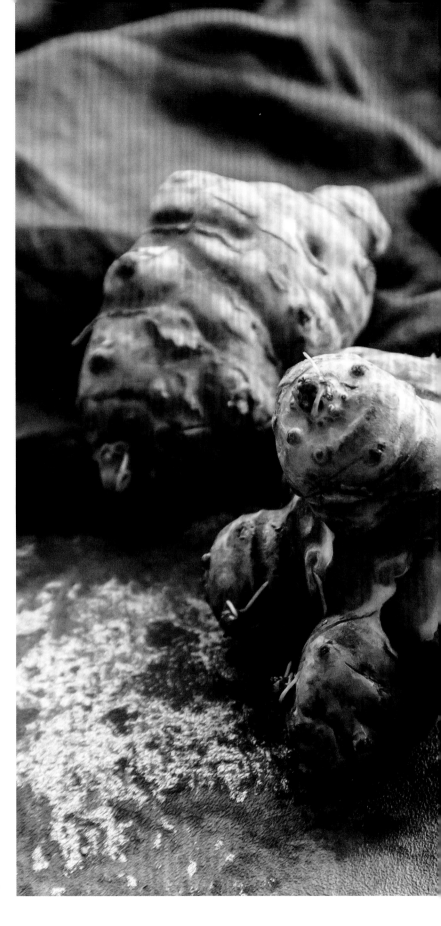

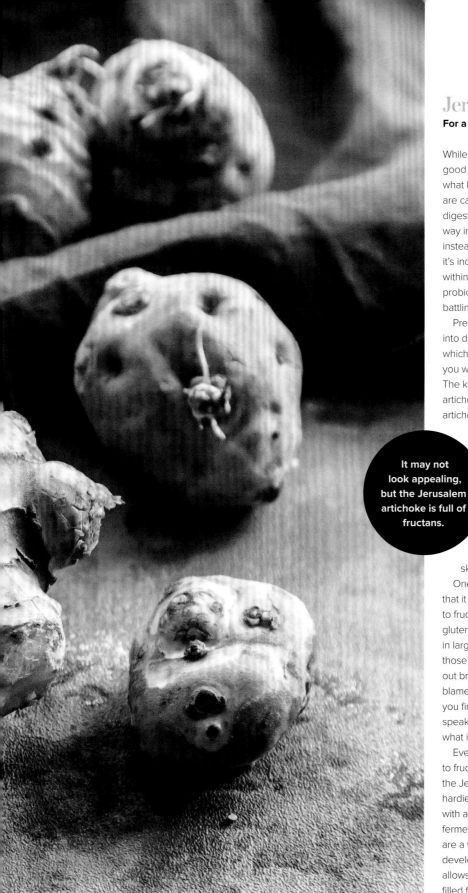

Jerusalem artichokes
For a feast of fructans

While probiotics are the source of the good bacteria in your gut, prebiotics are what keep them doing their job. These are carbohydrates that cannot be digested normally, so instead make their way into the gut where they ferment instead. It may not sound ideal, but in fact it's incredibly useful as fermentation within the gut provides fuel for the probiotics to keep on living, working and battling that bad bacteria.

Prebiotics can be broken down further into different groups and types, one of which is the fructan, a polymer that helps you with your regularity and digestion. The king of the fructan is the Jerusalem artichoke (which isn't actually an artichoke, rather a member of the sunflower family). Around 70 per cent of a Jerusalem artichoke is made up of fructans, so one will go a long way towards your recommended daily allowance. They also contain one-quarter of your recommended daily allowance of thiamin, which keeps your skin, hair and nails looking good.

One thing to be wary of, however, is that it is possible to have an intolerance to fructan that many people confuse for a gluten intolerance. Fructan can be found in large quantities in wheat, so when those suffering from bloating and gas cut out bread and feel better, they often blame the gluten instead of fructans. If you find yourself experiencing discomfort, speak to your doctor to find out exactly what is causing your problems.

Even if you don't have an intolerance to fructans, it is important not to overdo the Jerusalem artichoke as even the hardiest stomach can struggle to cope with all the gas created by the fermentation process. However, fructans are a vital part of the process towards developing a healthy gut, so if your body allows you, go to town on this fructan-filled flower.

> **It may not look appealing, but the Jerusalem artichoke is full of fructans.**

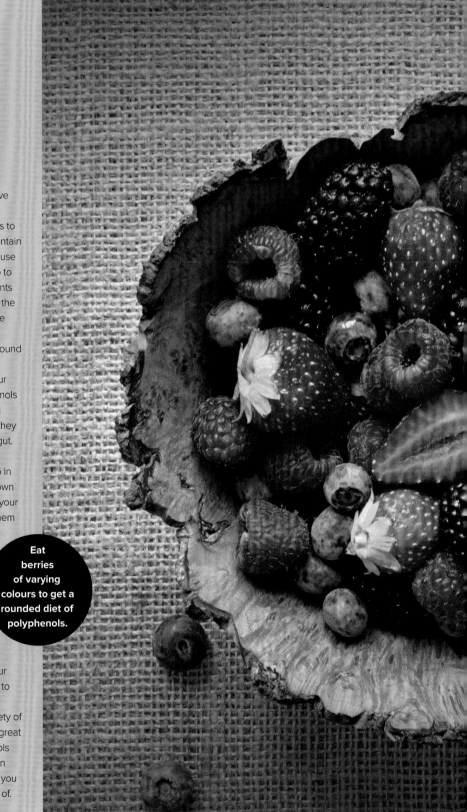

Berries

**Foods that are berry full
of polyphenols**

There's a good chance you'll have
heard of antioxidants. These are
molecules that attach themselves to
free radicals – molecules that contain
an unpaired electron and can cause
harm to the body. By hooking up to
these free radicals, the antioxidants
neutralise the threat and reduce the
risk of degenerative diseases like
cancer and dementia.

Polyphenols are compounds found
in plants that are packed full of
antioxidants, helping to keep your
body healthy. However, polyphenols
aren't just content with providing
large volumes of antioxidants – they
are also good friends with your gut.
As much as 95 per cent of the
polyphenols in your food end up in
your colon, where they break down
and have a prebiotic effect with your
gut's friendly bacteria, feeding them
and allowing them to multiply.
Elderberries, blackberries
and blueberries are
among the best in terms
of milligrams of
polyphenols per gram
and have the added
benefit of lowering your
cholesterol, while grapes fuel
the bacteria that strengthens your
intestinal wall, enabling your gut to
more easily fulfil its function.

We all know that eating a variety of
colourful fruit and vegetables is great
for our health, but the polyphenols
that feed bacteria and strengthen
your gut is an added bonus that you
should certainly take advantage of.

**Eat
berries
of varying
colours to get a
rounded diet of
polyphenols.**

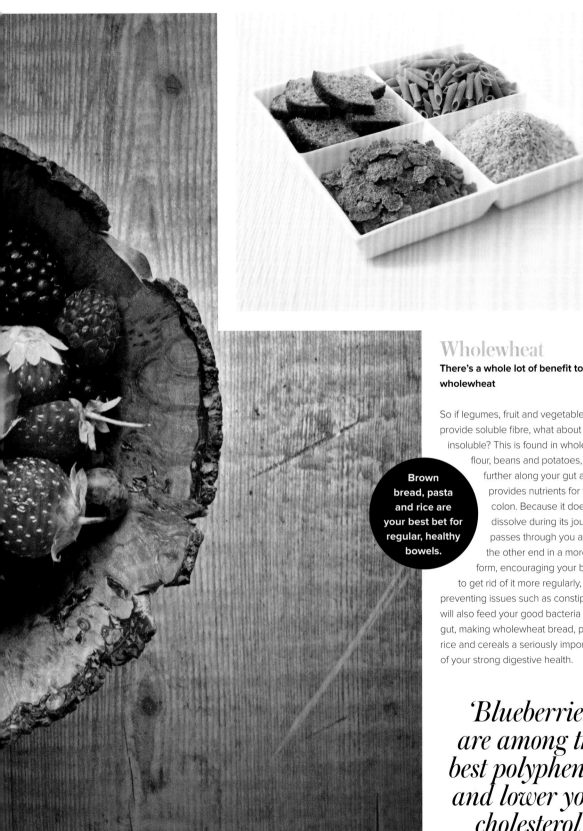

Wholewheat

There's a whole lot of benefit to wholewheat

So if legumes, fruit and vegetables provide soluble fibre, what about insoluble? This is found in wholewheat flour, beans and potatoes, travels further along your gut and provides nutrients for your colon. Because it doesn't dissolve during its journey, it passes through you and out the other end in a more solid form, encouraging your bowels to get rid of it more regularly, thus preventing issues such as constipation. It will also feed your good bacteria in your gut, making wholewheat bread, pasta, rice and cereals a seriously important part of your strong digestive health.

Brown bread, pasta and rice are your best bet for regular, healthy bowels.

'Blueberries are among the best polyphenols and lower your cholesterol'

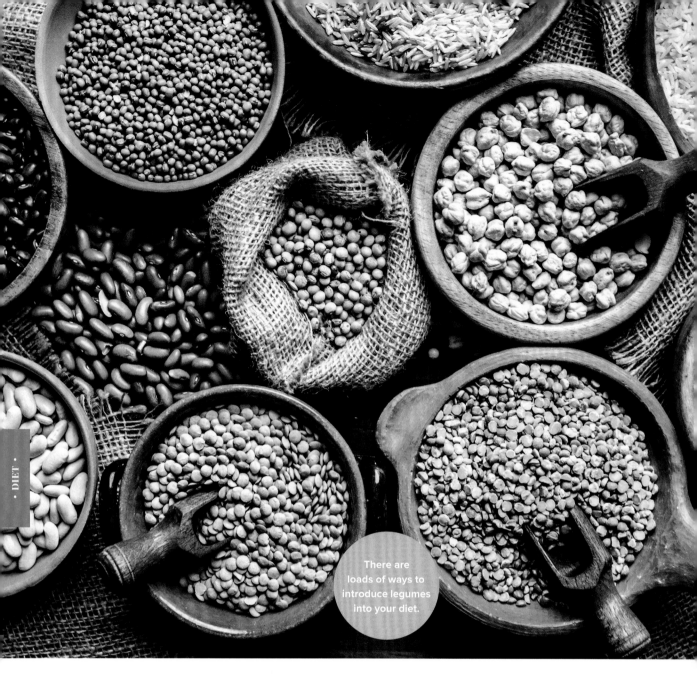

There are loads of ways to introduce legumes into your diet.

Legumes

A sure-fire way to more fibre

'Just half a cup of edamame beans contains 9g of fibre'

The other crucial element of good gut health is fibre. This is because fibre is what keeps your bowel movements regular, solid and soft. It can be found in large quantities in fruit, vegetables and carbohydrates. There are different types of fibre and all foods will offer different extra nutrients, so it is important you eat a range of foods to get as many different benefits as possible into your gut. Some people will also have intolerances, but

that means they'll just have to look elsewhere to find the fibre they need in their diet, and it's rare that they'd have to look far as fibre is abundant in natural foods. Soluble fibre is found in oranges, avocado and sweet potato, dissolves in water and aids digestion. Guidance suggests that the average adult should be eating around 30g of fibre per day, but most only get around 18g. An easy way to

increase the amount of fibre you get in your diet is to add legumes to your meals. The legume family covers most beans, chickpeas, lentils and peas. Just half a cup of edamame beans contains 9g of fibre, making it a quick way to up your intake. Adding chickpeas and lentils to your meal helps bulk up dinner, reduce the amount of meat you eat and provide healthy fibre and protein to your diet.

Red wine

Your evening tipple could be helping your gut

In a rare win for something being both delicious and good for you, it turns out that drinking red wine can aid your health. Grapes are naturally high in polyphenols, and therefore so is wine – with red out-polyphenoling white. A study showed that regular, but moderate, red wine drinkers had much better gut microbe diversity than those who drank white wine, beer, spirits or no alcohol at all. This improved diversity led to lower bad cholesterol and obesity in the subjects.

'Grapes are naturally high in polyphenols'

Yes, red wine is good for you. No, not the whole bottle.

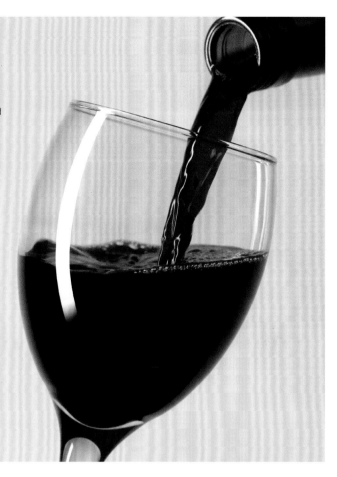

Cloves

The festive favourite packed with polyphenols

You may associate Christmas with turkey, mince pies, chocolates and hearing an elderly relative letting off a few unwelcome noises in front of the fire. Overeating is a big part of the festive season and that comes with its own, somewhat smelly, problems. That's where festive favourite cloves come into their own.

A study showed that cloves have more polyphenols and antioxidants than any other foodstuff, meaning that your mulled wine is fully loaded with health-giving chemicals, as well as tasting delicious. When ingested, cloves help the lining of your intestines relax, reducing the severity of any potential flatulence or diarrhoea that comes from that extra helping of Christmas pudding.

Cloves can save your Christmas in more ways than one.

The truth about
starchy
FOOD

We also know them as complex carbohydrates, but are starchy foods as unhealthy as we've been led to believe?

W live in an era that reveres high-protein, low-carb diets and demonises starch, but is it really better to abandon starchy foods, which many of us love? While it's true that consistently eating the wrong sort of starch can contribute to issues such as diabetes and weight gain, the right sort of starch is not only nutritious, but an excellent source of energy for both the body and brain. So, before ditching that baked potato or favourite sandwich, read on…

WHAT ARE STARCHES?

'They're our main source of carbohydrates and include foods such as potatoes, bread, rice, pasta, cereals and oats,' says Healthspan nutritionist Rob Hobson. 'According to government dietary advice, these foods should make up about a third of what we eat.' Starch can also be found in dairy products, fruits and vegetables, nuts, seeds and sugary treats.

ARE STARCHES GOOD FOR US?

According to the NHS, starches contain fibre, calcium and, gram for gram, fewer than half the calories of fat. 'Many starchy foods, especially cereals, are a good source of minerals including iron, zinc and magnesium,' says Rob. 'They're also an excellent source of B vitamins, helping the body to convert food into energy and maintain a healthy nervous system.'

However, not all starchy foods are created equally – refined carbs are 'made up of just one to two sugar molecules so the body can absorb and digest them more quickly and easily than unrefined starches,' says nutritionist Mays Al-Ali. 'This raises blood sugars much faster, but often causes an energy crash, leaving you tired and craving more.' It's this overeating of refined carbs, such as white bread, pizza dough and sweet desserts that leads to weight gain.

WORDS: DEB WATERS. PHOTOS: GETTY, ALAMY.
DR LAURE HYVERNAT (THENATURALCONSULTATION.COM). MAYS AL-ALI (HEALTHYMAYS.COM)

VITAL ROLE

According to the NHS, cutting carbs may cause...

✛ Digestive issues ✛ Dizziness
✛ Fatigue ✛ Headaches
✛ Irritability
✛ Nausea
✛ Sugar cravings

WHAT STARCH SHOULD I BE EATING?

Mays recommends aiming for fibre-rich, unrefined carbs – whole starches such as brown rice, wholewheat bread and pasta, legumes, nuts, seeds, cereals such as unprocessed oats and bran, and whole fruits and veg, plus sweet potato. As well being prized for their nutritional value, they take longer to digest and contribute to a lower risk of disease and better metabolic health. 'Whole and fibre-rich carbs are an amazing source of energy with a low glycaemic index, so they deliver energy in a controlled way and insulin peaks are avoided,' adds nutrition expert Dr Laure Hyvernat. 'Starches are also an essential prebiotic, feeding our guts with healthy bacteria. And they have a satiating effect that's helpful for sustainable weight management.'

Did you know?
There are fewer calories in resistant starches than normal starches, making them great for appetite control and weight management.

'Only 19% of adults in the UK eat the recommended 30g fibre per day,' says Rob. 'Fibre helps to reduce the risk of heart disease and bowel cancer.'

WHAT ABOUT RESISTANT STARCHES?

Resistant starches are indigestible, and function like a type of fibre. 'Because of this they end up in your colon where they act as prebiotics to feed bacteria, helping them to flourish,' says Rob. They help lower blood sugar levels after eating, reduce inflammation in the body and improve metabolic health, and may combat certain digestive issues. Research from the University of Colorado Denver also shows that resistant starches are especially beneficial for the colon and are linked to reduced risk of colorectal cancer.

WHERE CAN I FIND THEM?

Beans, peas, lentils, barley, sourdough and rye bread and plantains contain resistant starch. They also 'form on foods like potatoes, pasta, rice and oats once they've been cooked then cooled,' explains Rob. 'Brown rice works well as a cold salad base, or try making homemade sushi,' he adds. You can also reheat this food – just ensure you've cooled and stored everything correctly to avoid food poisoning.

WILL I PUT ON WEIGHT?

Carbs are an excellent source of energy, but when we eat more than our bodies need, or poor-quality refined carbs 'they promote storage of fat,' says Dr Hyvernat. 'That's why it's important to personalise our diets to our individual energy requirements.'

MAKE YOUR GUT HAPPY WITH THESE SIMPLE STARCH SWAPS...

SWAP...
- White bread
- White rice
- White pasta
- Fruit juice
- Processed cereals
- Chips and fries

FOR....
- Wholegrain or granary bread
- Brown or wild rice, or quinoa
- Wholewheat or bean pasta
- Whole fruit
- Unprocessed bran or oats
- Skin-on baked potatoes or home-made wedges

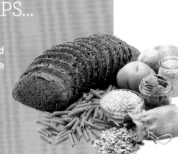

Secrets of a *HEALTHY* *store* CUPBOARD

Stock your cupboards with long-life
essentials so that you always have
something healthy to rustle up in the
absence of fresh food

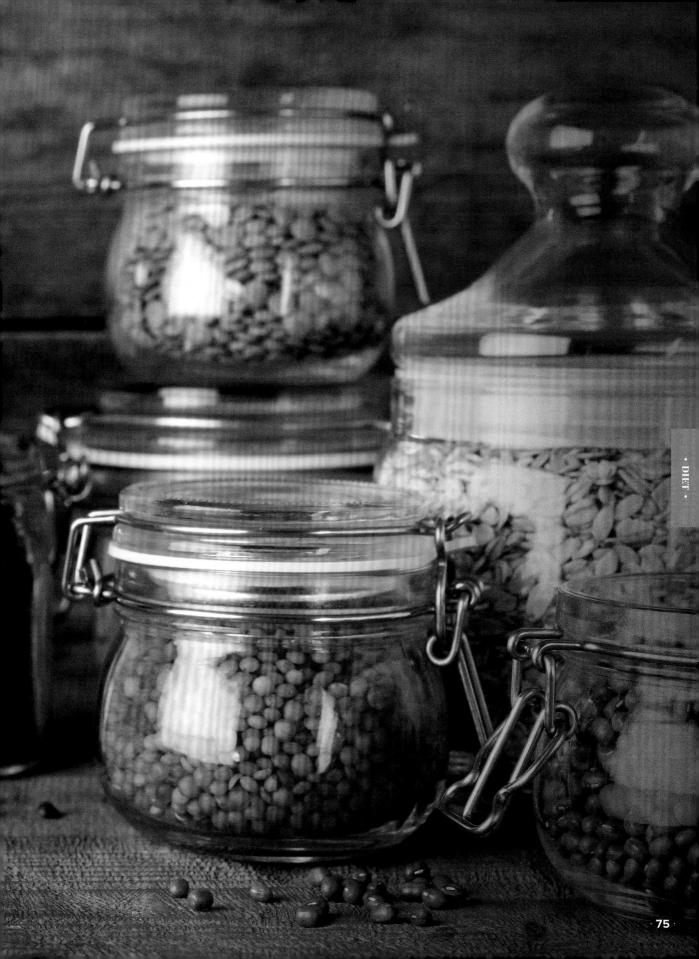

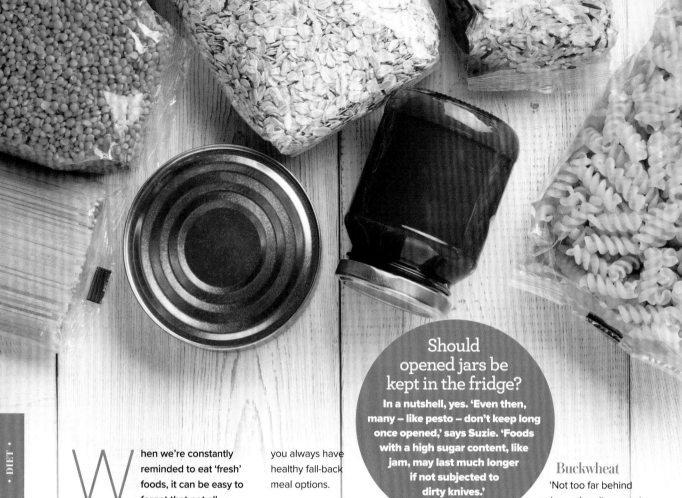

When we're constantly reminded to eat 'fresh' foods, it can be easy to forget that not all healthy food has to be fresh.

In the early days of the 2020 lockdown, when we were all avoiding supermarkets and facing food shortages, many of us had to rely largely on what we had in the store cupboard – and it turns out that this way of eating is not as unhealthy as it might at first sound – especially as it's reduced our reliance on over-priced ready meals and processed foods, and helped us get into the healthy habit of cooking from scratch.

While fresh produce, as we're frequently told, is often best, the foods we find in our pantries can be packed full of goodness, too.

If your cupboards are looking a little sparse, here's what to stock up on so you always have healthy fall-back meal options.

Quinoa

This ancient South American seed has become a nutrition buzzword for good reason: it contains fibre, protein and an abundance of nutrients.

'Three-quarters of a cup of quinoa contains around 8g of protein – double the equivalent of rice,' says Suzie Sawyer, clinical nutritionist and founder of Nutrition Lifestyle. 'It's also a great source of manganese, magnesium and zinc.'

It's gluten-free too, unlike wheat-based grains, such as couscous. It can taste a bit bland served on its own, but cooked in one-pot dishes like chilli or curry, it will take on the flavour of the sauce for a high-protein, filling meal.

Fresh fruit and veg sell-bys

'In the fridge or a dark cupboard or box, most fruit and veg can last past its sell-by date,' explains Suzie. 'Go by the colour and feel of the food instead.'

Should opened jars be kept in the fridge?

In a nutshell, yes. 'Even then, many – like pesto – don't keep long once opened,' says Suzie. 'Foods with a high sugar content, like jam, may last much longer if not subjected to dirty knives.'

Buckwheat

'Not too far behind quinoa when it comes to protein content, buckwheat is often mistaken for a seed, but is actually part of the rhubarb family. And, just like rhubarb, it's helpful for balancing hormones.

'Buckwheat has a high lignan content,' Suzie explains. 'Lignans are a class of phytoestrogens – naturally-occurring substances in food that have a positive oestrogen-like effect.'

Despite its name, buckwheat contains no wheat or gluten, but it is packed full of B vitamins, which are often lost during refining. Buckwheat flour is great for pancakes, or you can use it as the base for a tasty filling salad or in place of rice.

Cannellini beans

If you have a tin of these beans gathering dust, it's time to put them to good use.

'Cannellini beans are known as alpha amylase inhibitors, which means they help block the starch-digesting enzyme

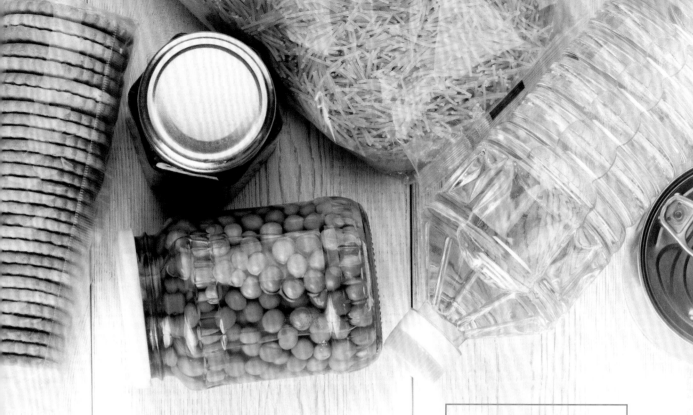

amylase, so foods are absorbed further down the digestive tract,' explains Suzie. 'This lowers their GI value, keeping blood-glucose in balance.'

They're are also high in protein, fibre, calcium and potassium. Add to salads, soups and pasta sauces to make them more filling.

Rolled oats

This breakfast staple is 100 per cent wholegrain and absolutely brilliant for keeping energy sustained throughout the morning.

'Rolled oats are full of fibre so are great for keeping bowels running super-smoothly,' says Suzie. 'They also contain a type of fibre called beta-glucan, which has been found to help lower cholesterol levels.'

A standard 40g serving of rolled oats with 300ml of semi skimmed milk contains 15g of protein – another reason

they'll keep you feeling fuller for longer. Be sure to stick to rolled, though; instant oats have had some fibre stripped away during processing.

Tinned tuna

'Government advice is to eat two portions of fish (one oily) weekly but, for most of us, consumption has remained consistently below these dietary recommendations,' says Suzie. 'Often this is because people are unsure how to cook fish – well, there's a meal in a can right here! Sardines and salmon also supply super-healthy omega-3 fats, essential for the heart, eyes, skin, hormones and joints.'

Tinned meat and fish can last around two to four years unopened. Once opened, keep leftovers in a sealed container in the fridge. For a simple meal, mash with olive oil and herbs, spread onto crusty bread and grill.

The shelf life of rice

Uncooked white rice can last for up to 20 years in an airtight container, despite the pack date! Be more wary of brown rice, as the oily bran and germ can go rancid.

THE FACTS ON FROZEN

Frozen fruit and veg make easy, nutrient-rich additions to meals – with no waste!

Despite the fresh-food hype, most frozen fruit and veg are frozen straight after harvest, so retain their nutrient content. 'Generally, frozen is as good as fresh,' says Suzie. 'In fact, often, fresh fruits and veg are stored for long periods before being sold, which reduces their nutrient content.

'The downside of frozen fruits and veg is that they're often sold "prepared". Any food preparation, including chopping or peeling, reduces nutrient content because much of it is found just under the skin.'

Most fruit and veg can be frozen for around 18 months. However, fresh meat and poultry that is then frozen only lasts around six months before drying out and losing taste.

Could
PROBIOTICS
CHANGE YOUR LIFE?

Everything from mood to heart health can be linked back to
our gut – so it's time we started taking care of it...

Not familiar with pro and prebiotics? That's about to change. Because these supplements could play a pivotal role in our health. While you probably only think about your gut health when you have stomach pains or indigestion, scientists are learning that bacteria teeming in our guts play a vital role throughout our bodies. Some are beneficial, helping digestion, for example, others are neutral and some very unhelpful.

Your microbiome – the community of microbes living in your gut – is unique to you. Unfortunately, the typical Western lifestyle – low-fibre diet, antibiotics, excessive hygiene and high stress levels – isn't bacteria friendly, which is where the pro and pre supplements come in...

PROBIOTICS

Probiotics – healthy live bacteria – can do us a world of good. 'Live bacteria supplements have been shown to help support the health of the gut lining, reducing the risk of leaky gut or gut hyper-permeability, thought to contribute to numerous inflammatory conditions,' says Hannah Braye, nutritional therapist at Bio-Kult (bio-kult.com). 'Having a healthy gut lining is also important for the absorption of nutrients from food. As over 70 per cent of immune cells are located in the gut and communicate directly with our gut bacteria, evidence also indicates that live bacteria supplements help our ability to fight infections. Many people also don't realise that our gut bacteria aids detoxification processes, and that live bacteria supplements help bind toxins in the gut, and can be of benefit in conditions such as non-alcoholic fatty liver disease.'

Probiotics also benefit your wellbeing. 'How the balance of bacteria in the gut can effect mental health is an exciting and rapidly evolving area of research, with the use of live bacteria supplements showing great promise.'

PREBIOTICS

'While probiotics are the live bacteria, the less-known prebiotics are what feed the good bacteria, helping them thrive – like a fertiliser for your own gut flora,' says Glenn Gibson, professor of Food Microbiology at the University of Reading. 'A growing body of research suggests prebiotics might benefit everything from our mood and sleep to immunity and obesity.'

'Although prebiotics are found in onions, garlic and leeks, in order to experience meaningful health benefits, you would have to eat unrealistically large amounts. Taking a prebiotic supplement, is a more convenient way of boosting immunity.'

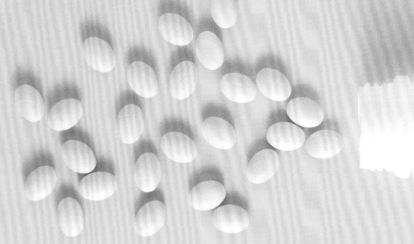

REAP THE REWARDS

A happy gut and varied gut bacteria can prove beneficial for many things...

MOOD Scientists sometimes call the gut the "second brain" – because of the theory that bugs living there can affect mental health. Research from the APC Microbiome Institute at University College Cork found low levels of gut microbes raised the risk of anxiety and depression, while higher amounts of bugs lowered it.

COLON CANCER RISK

Research from the Dana-Farber Cancer Institute in the US has found that a bacteria called f.nucleatum contributes to the development of many colon tumours – and having a diverse microbiome may help control this effect.

WEIGHT A French study found people with lots of different healthy bacteria living in their gut were more likely to be slim, while those with lower levels have a higher risk of obesity.

DIGESTION 'IBS, with symptoms including bloating and constipation, and/or diarrhoea, is often linked with low-diversity gut bugs,' says author and professor of genetics Tim Spector, author of *The Diet Myth*. Research shows some strains of bacteria help ease symptoms of IBS, which may partly be down to the effect they have on stress chemicals involved in the condition.

ALLERGIES

Suffering from hay fever, eczema or asthma? Low levels of gut bugs may be to blame. A US-led study published in the journal *Nature Medicine* found less diverse gut bugs may be linked with a higher chance of developing asthma and other allergies. Meanwhile, a US review of studies found taking probiotics could lower your risk of hay fever.

AGEING 'In a study, when we transplanted poo from younger fish into older ones, they lived longer – so microbes seem to have an important anti-ageing role,' says Professor Spector. Thankfully, unlike those fish, you don't need a faecal transplant to stay youthful, but boosting your bugs could help slow the ageing process.

HEART HEALTH Studies have found people with a certain group of gut bugs, called collinsella, are more likely to have hardened arteries. It's thought to do with the way the bacteria interact with certain foods, triggering the release of chemicals that cause arterial stiffening. Danish research found having low levels of bacteria in your gut could make you more prone to inflammation in your arteries, raising heart disease risk.

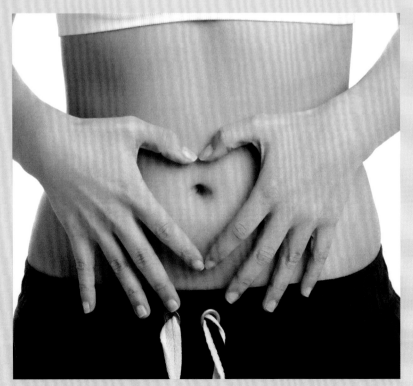

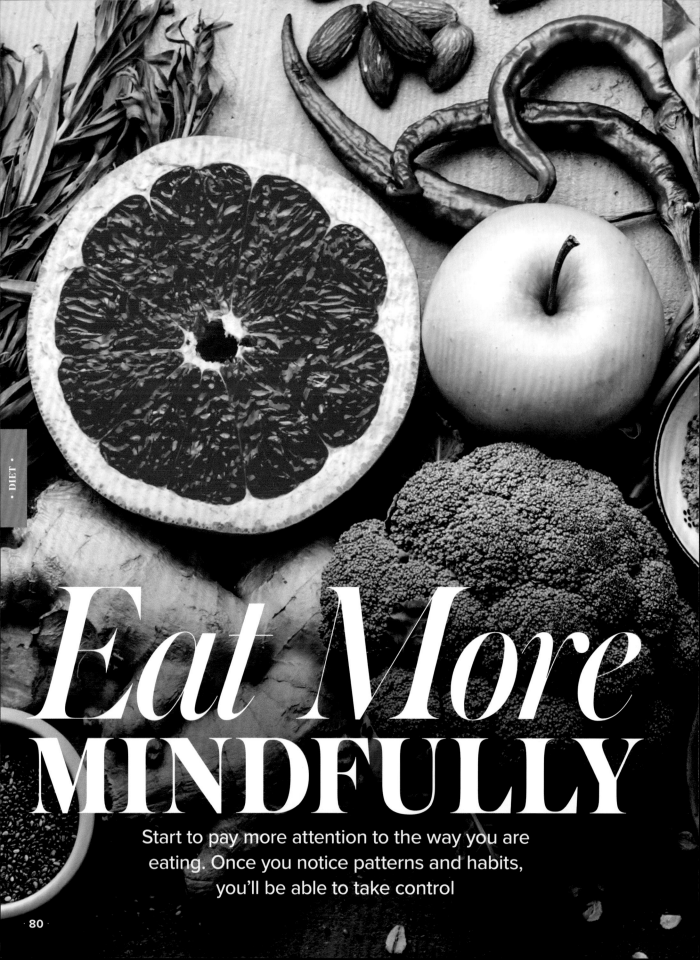

Eat More MINDFULLY

Start to pay more attention to the way you are
eating. Once you notice patterns and habits,
you'll be able to take control

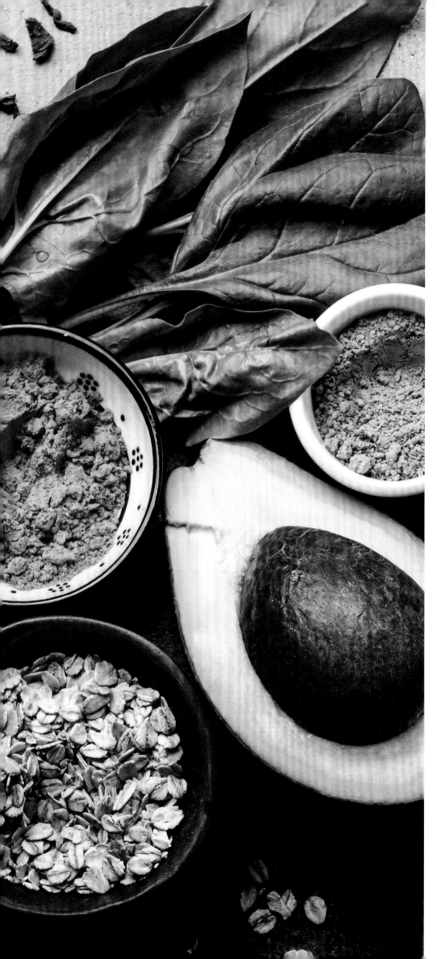

indful eating is about paying attention at the time of eating and noticing what you're thinking, feeling and eating through all five senses. It's about being conscious of your eating behaviour – what you're doing and when you're doing it. Think of it as the polar opposite to eating on autopilot.

By paying more attention to these things moment by moment, we can start to make conscious choices about what we're eating, and make wiser decisions that will help us in achieving health and fitness goals. The concept of good or bad food doesn't exist in a mindful eating approach. It's about viewing food as fuel and therefore consuming energy to enable us to function throughout the day. Different fuel is of course helpful for different things, and mindful eating isn't about being perfect all the time; rather it enables you to be in a state where you can make conscious decisions about what to eat.

BENEFITS OF MINDFUL EATING

Mindful eating can give you a route to happiness that's enduring. Happiness doesn't come from the external stuff like cars, houses or being a certain weight. It comes from within, from your own experience of acceptance, self-compassion, non-judgement and knowing you're in control. Therefore if you can nurture your internal experience, you're not having to abuse your body or relationship with food to feel a sense of worth. Other benefits include:

✛ It can flush out whether you're an emotional eater rather than eating when you're actually hungry. You can then start to tackle the root cause of your emotional distress and manage your emotions better instead of blocking them out and smothering them with food.

✛ It can be empowering to know that you are in control rather than making emotional food choices.

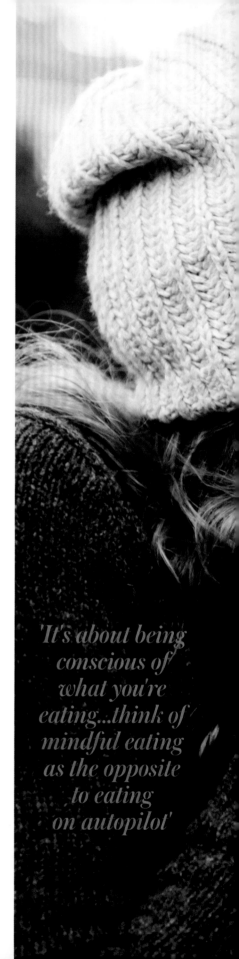

✤ It can change your relationship with food as you start making wiser choices about what you eat.

✤ It can give you liberation and freedom from food's mercy and fear of food.

✤ It's a long-term lifestyle change and can be an alternative approach to following a restrictive or quick-fix diet.

✤ If you can start to view food as fuel, you'll recognise when you're eating in ways that are not supporting your healthy behaviour.

✤ It can reduce binge eating as you simply cannot eat in this way if you're being mindful. The more you develop being mindful, you can start to intercept binge-eating behaviour or learn to stop it before it starts. Through mindful eating, you begin to recognise the triggers, the thoughts and feelings that are happening so you can stop and then make a choice about how to proceed.

DEVELOPING THE SKILL OF MINDFUL EATING OVER TIME

So how long will it take for you to start feeling the impact and benefits of eating mindfully? And how often should you ideally be practising to develop the trait or skill of mindfulness? Unfortunately, this is a difficult question to answer because there are many factors at play, such as the amount of times per day/week of practising, the quality of the practice, and the individual's propensity to learn. Just like learning to drive, we all take different amounts of time to learn new skills.

Recent research in workplaces where mindfulness is being trained and practised has identified benefits from practising ten minutes or more a day over an eight-week period. Psychologists argue on the length of time it takes to develop new habits, but most think it's between 30 and 90 days.

This is a great starting point for practising your mindful eating, and you should start to see benefits after eight to 12 weeks if you're practising for at least ten minutes a day. But view mindful eating as a lifestyle change and an ongoing commitment. Training and rewiring your brain is just like training your body to change; it takes time and requires continual attention and practice. Just as with exercise, you might face a relapse where you've got a really busy period at work, with no time to prepare healthy food, so you grab a sandwich at lunch and a takeaway for dinner. That turns into two or three days and you forget the importance of healthy eating or your mindful-eating practice, so everything takes a downward spiral. It's okay! We're human beings and life happens, so don't judge yourself and beat yourself up. Show yourself some compassion, treat yourself like you would your best friend and just start again when you can. Explore what triggered you to stop so you can watch out for those signs in the future. Recruiting a friend to help and support you is always really helpful – someone you can rely on and who will give you moral support when these difficult times happen.

TELL-TALE SIGNS THAT YOU MIGHT NOT BE EATING MINDFULLY

✤ You have a lack of awareness about your eating behaviour in all forms – what it is you're eating, when and why you're eating.

✤ You especially lack awareness of why you're eating, because this can link to your relationship with food and your emotions.

✤ You don't remember what you've eaten all day.

✤ You finish a chocolate bar (or other foods) without even noticing what it tasted like.

✤ You get to the end of the day and realise that you haven't had one proper meal; you've just been absent-mindedly grazing and snacking throughout the day instead.

✤ You recognise that your behaviours are out of sync with other people's, maybe eating in private or not eating anything at all.

✤ You're fearful of foods.

✤ You eat when you're not hungry.

'It's about being conscious of what you're eating...think of mindful eating as the opposite to eating on autopilot'

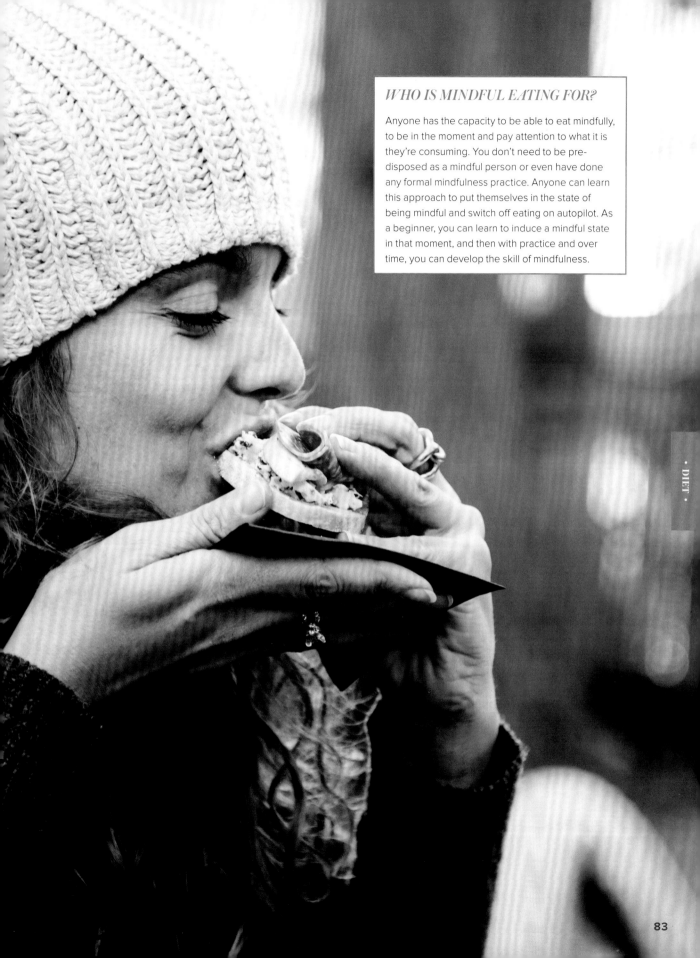

WHO IS MINDFUL EATING FOR?

Anyone has the capacity to be able to eat mindfully, to be in the moment and pay attention to what it is they're consuming. You don't need to be pre-disposed as a mindful person or even have done any formal mindfulness practice. Anyone can learn this approach to put themselves in the state of being mindful and switch off eating on autopilot. As a beginner, you can learn to induce a mindful state in that moment, and then with practice and over time, you can develop the skill of mindfulness.

Recipes

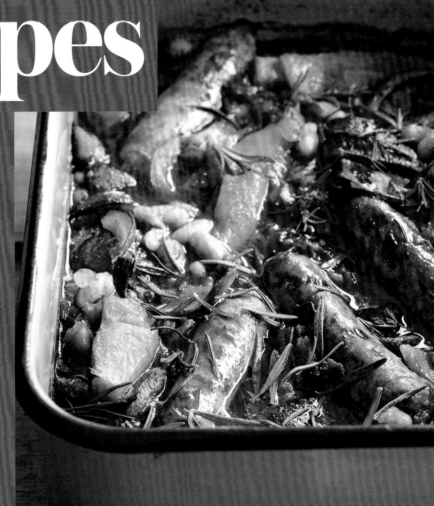

101

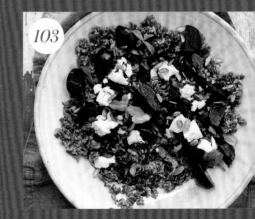

103

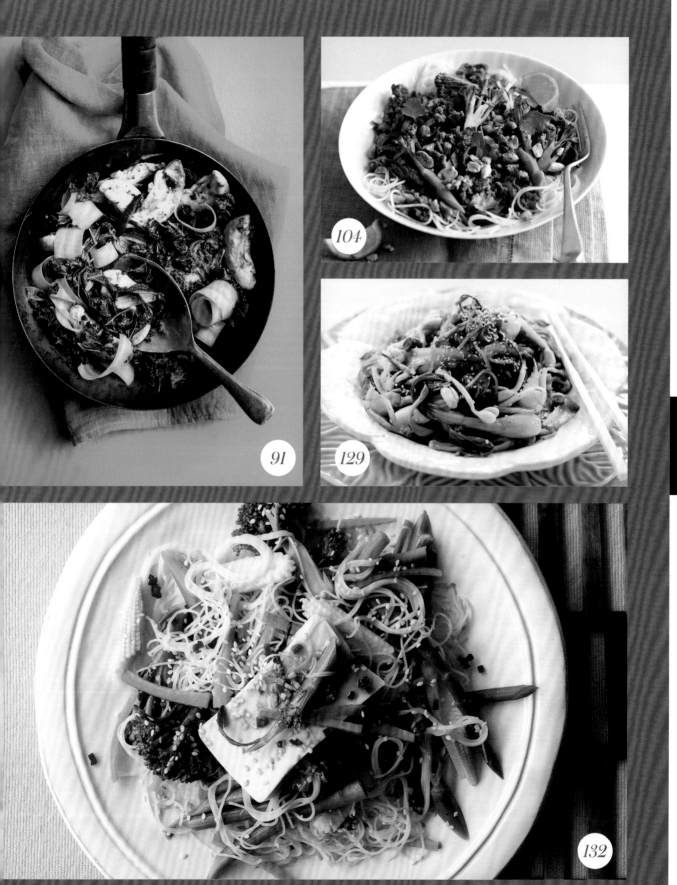

91

104

129

132

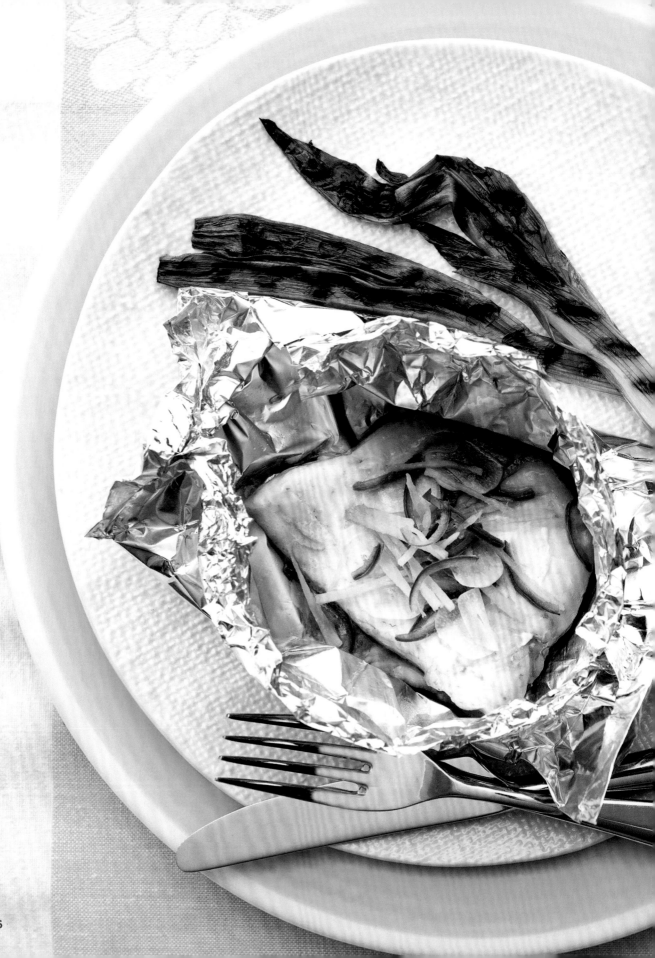

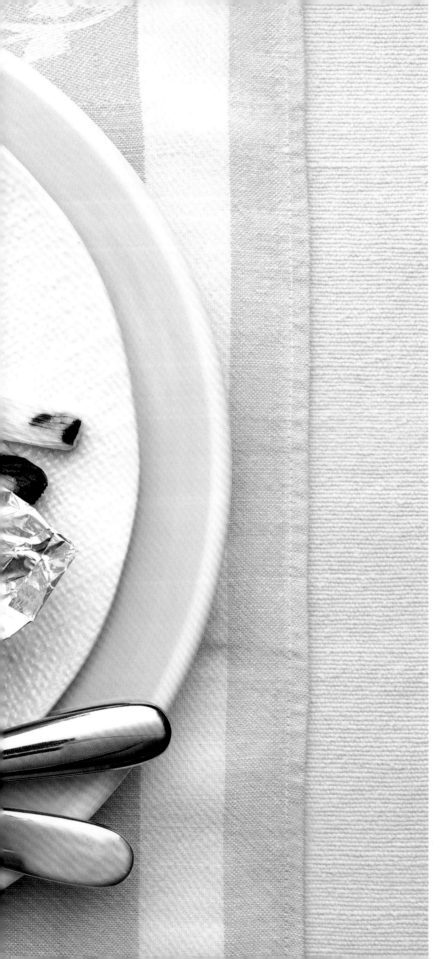

Soy and ginger steamed sea bass

Ginger root has long been used for medicinal purposes and can help if you're suffering from sinus congestion, as well as other ailments.

Serves: 1 • 20 mins

- **75g (2.6oz) skinless and boneless sea bass fillet**
- **1tsp finely sliced fresh root ginger**
- **½ green chilli, deseeded and finely sliced**
- **1 garlic clove, finely sliced**
- **1tsp dark soy sauce**
- **¼tsp sesame oil**
- **2 trimmed spring onions, halved**

1 Preheat the oven to 180°C/355°F/Gas 4. Place the sea bass fillet in the centre of a large piece of kitchen foil and scatter over the finely sliced ginger, green chilli and garlic. Drizzle over the dark soy sauce and sesame oil and fold over the foil, scrunching the edges together tightly to form a parcel. Place on a tray and bake for 10-12 mins, until the fish is cooked and aromatic.
2 Meanwhile, heat a ridged griddle pan and griddle the spring onions for 2-3 mins, turning occasionally, until nicely charred. Remove and set aside.
3 To serve, open the steamed sea bass parcel and then top with the griddled spring onions.

Onion bhajis

Onions contain the plant flavonol quercetin, which studies show can ease hay fever symptoms. 'Turmeric is proven to be anti-inflammatory,' adds Rob Hobson.

Makes: 8-10 bhajis • 30 mins

- **6tbsp plain flour**
- **1tsp turmeric**
- **1tsp ground cumin**
- **1tsp garam masala**
- **Salt**
- **2 onions, peeled and sliced**
- **Oil, for deep frying**
- **Raita (minty yoghurt), to serve**

1 In a bowl, mix together the flour, turmeric, cumin, garam masala and a little salt. Add 3-4tbsp water to make a stiff batter. Stir the sliced onions into the batter, to coat.

2 Heat the oil in a deep frying pan to 190°C/375°F (use a thermometer). Add 1tsp of the onion mixture to the pan. When it rises to the surface, add the next spoonful. Continue doing this until the pan is full.

3 Cook for 3-4 mins, turning the bhajis over halfway through, until cooked. Remove from the pan with a slotted spoon and drain them on kitchen paper.

4 Cook the remainder of the onion mixture in the same way, keeping the cooked bhajis warm. They can be served immediately, or reheated on a baking sheet in a hot oven for a few mins. Serve with raita, for dipping.

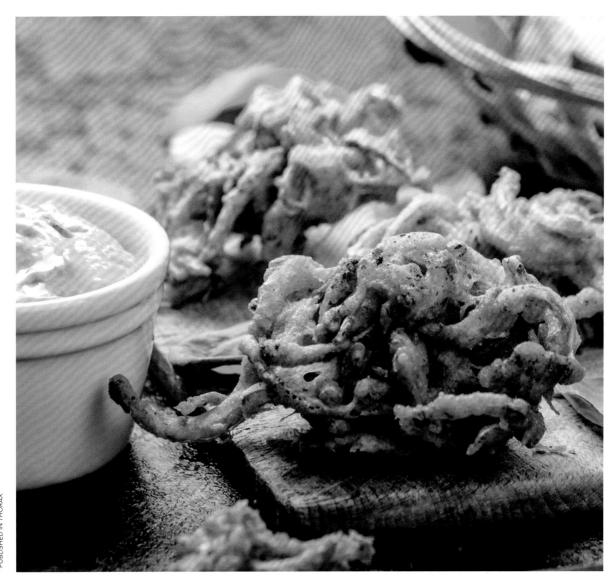

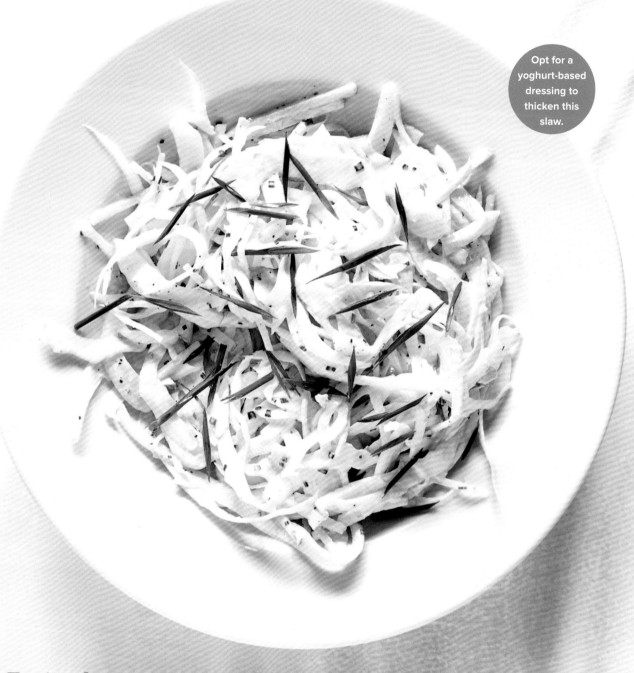

Opt for a yoghurt-based dressing to thicken this slaw.

Fruity slaw

Studies have suggested that apples may help protect against asthma.* This recipe gives you a crunch of one of your five-a-day alongside some digestion-friendly fennel.

Serves: 8-10 • 10 mins

- **1 green apple, cored, and cut into matchsticks**
- **1 fennel bulb, halved, very thinly sliced**
- **1 small white cabbage, very thinly sliced**
- **Juice of 1 lemon**
- **1tbsp white wine vinegar**
- **2tbsp finely chopped chives**
- **Home-made dressing**

1 Mix the apple, fennel and cabbage with the lemon juice and vinegar and set aside for 5 minutes to soften slightly. Add the chopped chives and dressing, mix well and season.

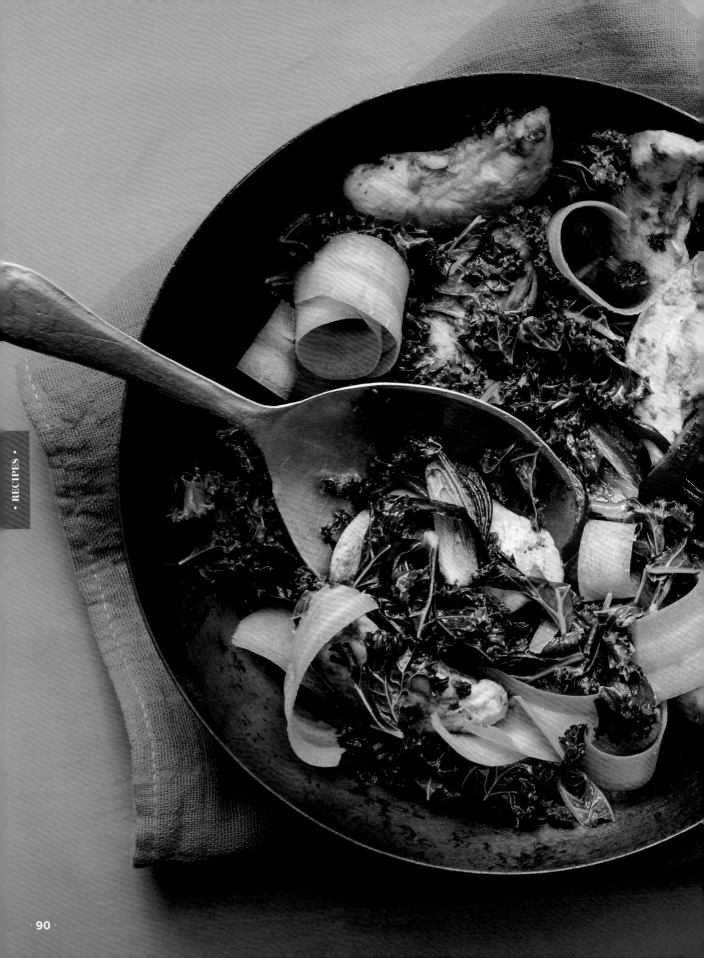

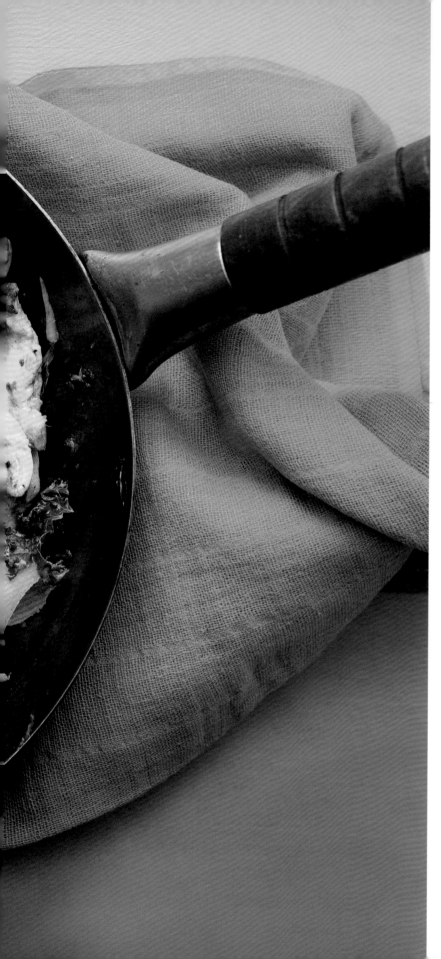

Chicken and kale stir-fry

Studies have found that the curcumin in turmeric appears to elevate serotonin levels, whilst lowering cortisol, a stress hormone.**

Serves 4 • 25 mins

- **425g (15oz) mini chicken breast fillets, or regular sized fillets sliced into smaller pieces**
- **2.5cm (1in) root ginger, peeled, grated**
- **2 garlic cloves, grated**
- **1 lemon, grated zest and juice**
- **2tbsp rapeseed oil**
- **¼tsp turmeric**
- **2 red onions, sliced**
- **250g (8.8oz) curly kale, chopped**
- **1tbsp miso paste**
- **2 carrots, peeled**

1 Put chicken into a shallow dish and season. Sprinkle over ginger, garlic and lemon zest. Squeeze on the lemon juice and stir to mix evenly.
2 Heat oil in a wok and fry the chicken for 3 mins without stirring. Sprinkle with the turmeric, turn and cook for 3 more mins.
3 Push the chicken to the side and add onions. Cook for 3 mins. Add the kale. Stir miso into 200ml (7fl oz) boiling water and add, cover and cook for 3 mins.
4 Use a peeler on the carrots to create ribbons. Add to the wok for 2 mins. Serve with quinoa.

**JOURNAL OF AFFECTIVE DISORDERS

Salmon Provençale with freekeh

Research has shown that omega-3 rich fatty fish such as salmon has a strong relationship with mental health, with one study*** finding that those whose diet lacked omega-3 increased their risk of developing mood disorders, such as anxiety.

Serves 4 • 30 mins

- 4 x 100g (3.5oz) pieces salmon fillet
- 250g (8.8oz) mixed tomatoes, larger ones quartered
- 2 garlic cloves, sliced
- 50g (1.8oz) mixed pitted olives
- 12 caper berries
- 1 lemon, sliced plus the juice of 1 lemon
- 100ml (3.4fl oz) dry white wine
- 2 x 250g (8.8oz) pouches cooked freekeh (such as Merchant Gourmet)
- Large handful mixed fresh herbs (parsley, coriander and basil), finely chopped

1 Heat oven to 200°C/390°F/Gas 6. Cut four 22cm (8.7in) circles of baking paper. Place a piece of salmon on one half of each circle. Add tomatoes, garlic, olives and caper berries, season and top with lemon slices. Place on a baking tray and pour wine into each parcel.

2 Fold and twist edges of each circle to seal. Bake in oven for 15 mins.

3 Heat freekeh following pack instructions. Add herbs and lemon juice and stir. Serve with the salmon.

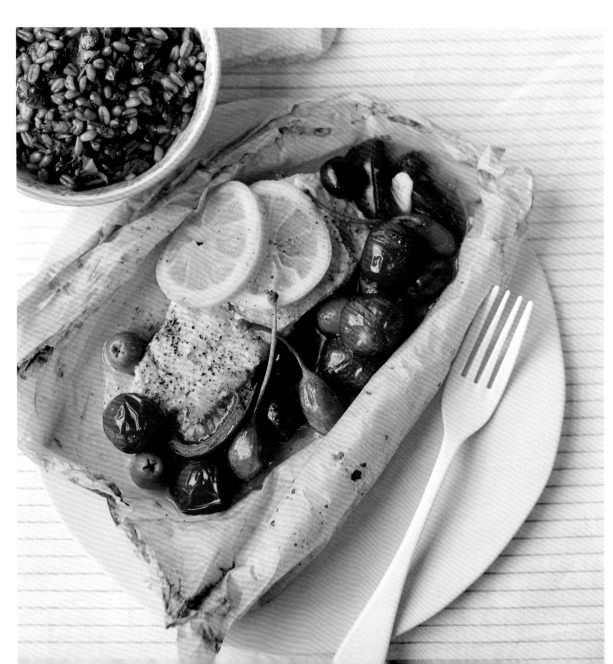

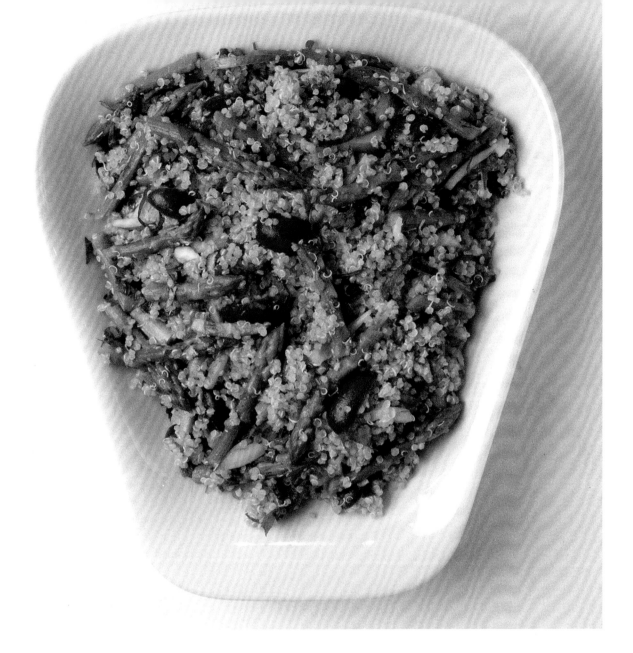

Quinoa and asparagus tabbouleh

Quinoa is a good source of magnesium and B vitamins. 'These are needed to produce anti-anxiety brain chemicals such as GABA (gamma-aminobutyric acid),' says Wild Nutrition founder, Henrietta Norton. 'Use quinoa as an alternative to rice or wheat pasta for managing anxiety and stress.'

Serves 4 · 35 mins

- **200g (7oz) quinoa**
- **2 bunches of asparagus, chopped into 4-5cm (2in) chunks**
- **150g (5.3oz) small tomatoes (such as cherry or plum), quartered**
- **1 red onion, finely sliced**
- **1 bunch fresh flat-leaf parsley, very finely chopped**
- **1 small handful fresh mint, very finely chopped**
- **2tbsp olive oil**
- **2tbsp lemon juice**

1 Cook the quinoa according to the instructions on the packet. Meanwhile, in a separate pan, simmer the asparagus for 2 mins. Drain and set aside.

2 Add the tomatoes, onion, parsley, mint, asparagus and the quinoa to a large bowl.

3 Add the olive oil and lemon juice to the bowl, then season well. Toss everything together and serve.

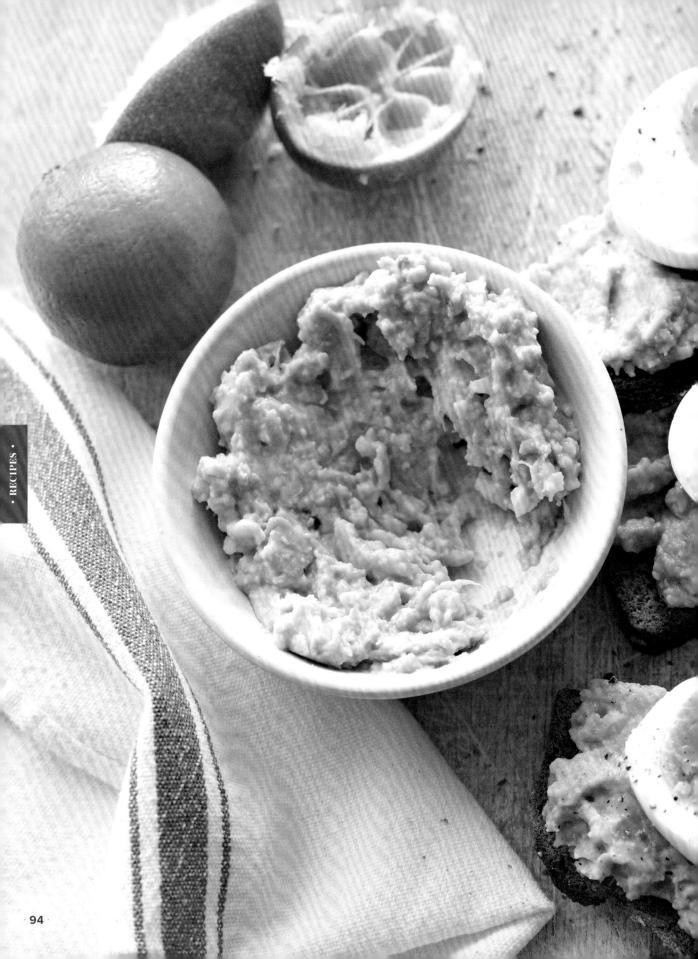

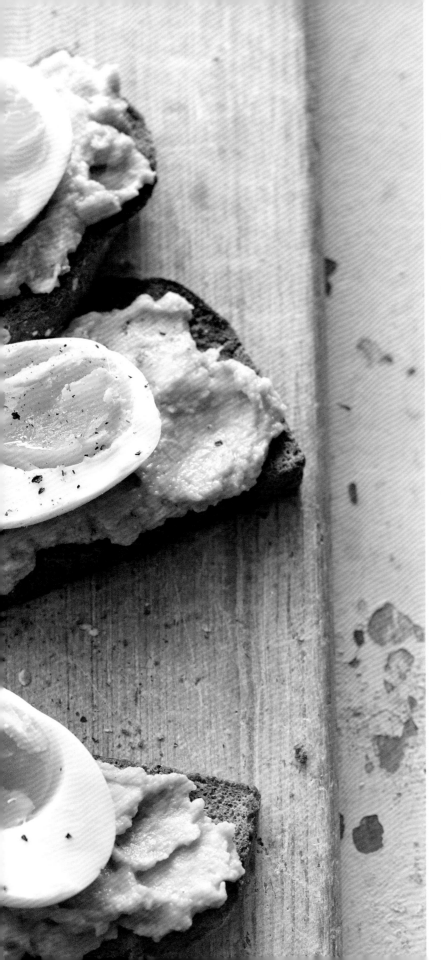

Smashed avo toast with soft-boiled eggs

Eggs are protein-rich and one of the few foods that contain vitamin D. This dish will banish mid-morning munchies, too.

Serves 4 • 10 mins

- **4 eggs**
- **2 avocados**
- **Juice of half a lime**
- **8 slices of soda bread**

1 Boil eggs in a pan of hot water for 7 mins to give a lightly-set centre. Meanwhile, stone avocados and peel and quarter them.
2 Put avocado flesh in a bowl and season generously. Squeeze over lime juice and mash well with a fork.
3 Toast soda bread slices and peel eggs.
4 Spread mashed avocado on the toast, halve the eggs then sit them on top.

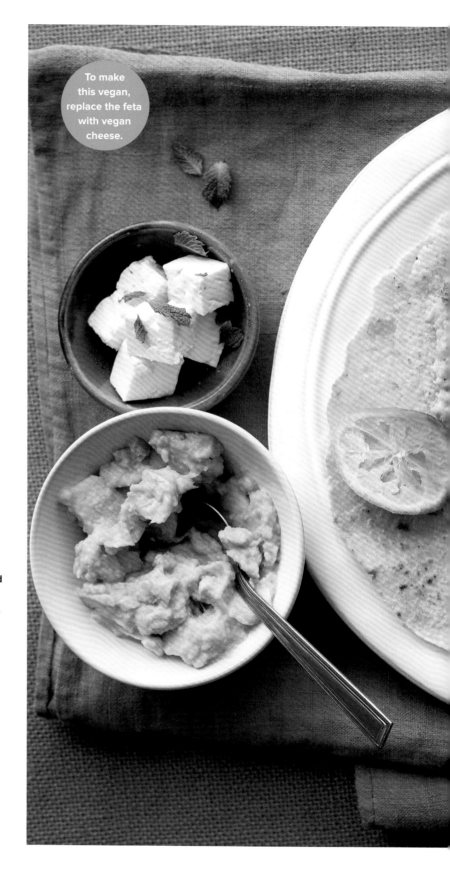

To make this vegan, replace the feta with vegan cheese.

Peri-peri rainbow wrap

Bursting with colourful veg, this healthy meal is quick to make.

Serves 2 • 25 mins

- Olive oil spray
- 400g (14oz) can black-eyed beans, drained and rinsed
- 1tsp peri-peri seasoning
- 1 avocado, stoned, peeled and chopped
- Juice of ½ lime
- 2 wholemeal or corn tortilla wraps
- 150g (5.3oz) red cabbage, shredded
- 1 large carrot, grated
- ⅓ cucumber, cut into julienne strips
- 4 radishes, quartered
- 100g (3.5oz) feta
- Few sprigs of mint
- 75g (2.6oz) beetroot, cut in wedges

1 Spray a non-stick pan with oil and gently fry the beans and peri-peri seasoning for 10 mins until crispy.
2 Mash the avocado with the lime juice.
3 Warm the wraps according to pack instructions and spread with avocado.
4 Combine cabbage, carrot, cucumber and radishes, then stir in the beans. Pile on top of the tortillas, sprinkle over the feta, mint and beetroot to serve.

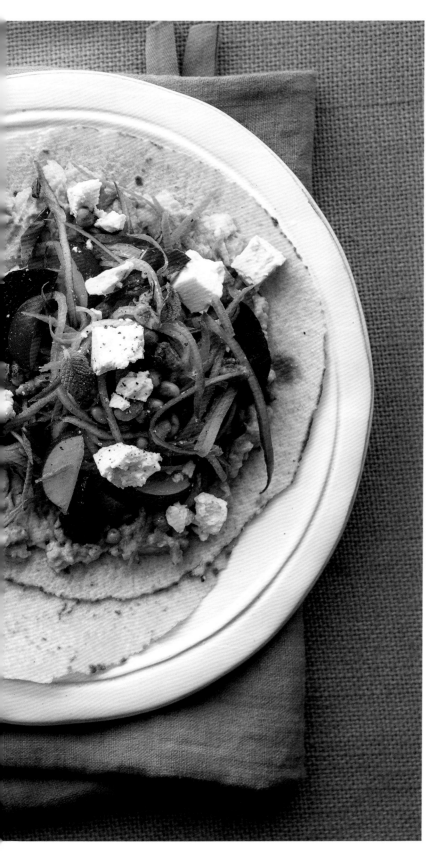

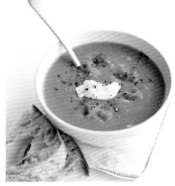

Spicy red pepper and lentil soup

This comforting soup is packed with vitamin C from the peppers, protein from the lentils and an immune-system boost from the garlic and chillies.

Serves 4 • 35-40 mins

- 200g (7oz) red lentils
- 2tbsp olive oil
- 1 medium onion, finely chopped
- 2 garlic cloves, peeled and crushed
- 1tsp crushed chillies
- 1tsp hot smoked paprika
- 4 red peppers, deseeded and diced
- 1l (2pt) vegetable stock
- 1tbsp sherry vinegar
- 1tsp caster sugar
- 4tbsp natural yoghurt

1 Rinse red lentils, then leave to soak in cold water. Meanwhile, in a large pan, warm olive oil and fry onion until soft. Add garlic and red chilli for 2 mins, then add sweet smoked paprika for a final minute with a splash of water.

2 Add red peppers and cover for 10 mins, stirring occasionally. Drain lentils, add to the pan with the vegetable stock, cover, bring to the boil and simmer for 15 mins until lentils begin to break down.

3 Reserve a third of the soup and blend the rest. Stir back into the chunky soup, season to taste adding the sherry vinegar and caster sugar. Divide between 4 bowls and swirl 1tbsp natural yoghurt through each.

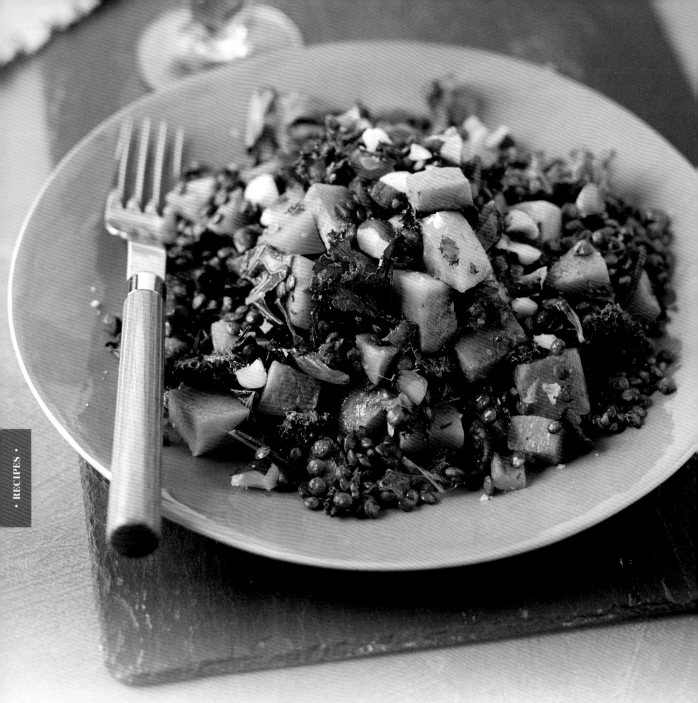

Lentil and roasted vegetable pilaf

Kale is a nutrient-dense food containing binding resins that can lower cholesterol levels. It's also a source of vitamins A, K and C, great for your immune system and vision.

Serves 4 • 25 mins

500g (17.6oz) butternut squash, cubed
1 garlic clove, crushed

2 red onions, chopped
1tbsp olive oil
300g (10.5oz) puy lentils
900ml (2pt) vegetable stock
175g (6.2oz) kale
60g (2oz) Brazil nuts

1 Preheat the oven to 200°C/390°F/ Gas 6. Spread the cubed squash over a roasting tin. Season and sprinkle with the garlic, red onions and oil. Roast for 20 mins.

2 Meanwhile, put the lentils and vegetable stock into a pan. Simmer gently for 20 mins, until just tender.

3 Stir the roasted squash, add the kale and Brazil nuts to the tin, and cook for just 3 mins, to crisp up the kale slightly.

4 Drain the lentils and tip into the roasting tray. Stir to combine, then serve.

Fresh blueberry yoghurt with maple syrup and golden oats

Oats contain beta-glucan, a soluble dietary fibre that's been shown to help lower cholesterol, while blueberries contain a chemical compound called pterostilbene as well as helpful antioxidant properties.

Serves 1 • 10 mins

- **Small handful rolled oats**
- **1tsp maple syrup**
- **15 blueberries, lightly crushed**
- **100g (3.5oz) fat-free natural yoghurt**

1 Start by dry-toasting the oats in a small frying pan over a medium heat, stirring frequently to prevent burning, for 6-8 mins, until pale golden and crisp. Tip out onto a plate to cool.

2 Drizzle ½tsp maple syrup into the bottom of a small glass tumbler. Quickly fold the blueberries into the yoghurt, reserving a few, and spoon onto the maple syrup.

3 Sprinkle the toasted oats on top, scatter over the reserved berries and drizzle with the remaining maple syrup.

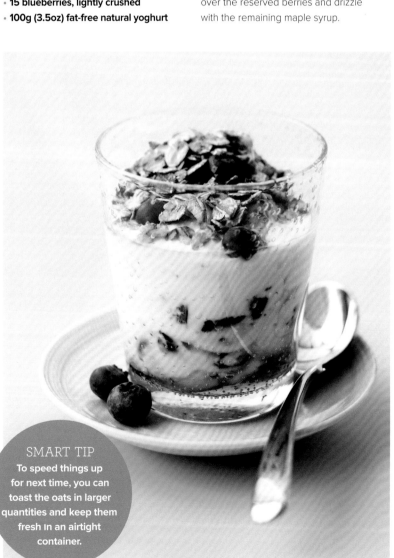

SMART TIP
To speed things up for next time, you can toast the oats in larger quantities and keep them fresh in an airtight container.

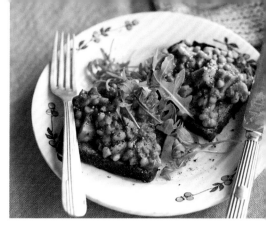

Homemade bumper baked beans on toast

Beans and pulses are rich in soluble fibre and can reduce your 'bad' cholesterol levels by up to five per cent according to one study***. Try to eat at least one portion a day – which is easy with this quick and tasty dish.

Serves 2 • 25 mins

- **125g (4.4oz) sweet potato, peeled and cubed**
- **¼tsp chipotle paste (or 1 pinch paprika)**
- **3tbsp tomato ketchup**
- **2tbsp malt vinegar**
- **1tbsp Worcestershire sauce**
- **1tsp honey**
- **1 celery stick, sliced**
- **400g (14oz) can haricot beans, drained and rinsed**
- **4 slices of wholemeal bread**
- **A handful of rocket**
- **Olive oil, to drizzle (optional)**

1 Put the sweet potato in a microwaveable bowl with 1tbsp water. Cook on high for 6 mins, until tender. (Alternatively, cook in boiling, salted water for 10 mins.)

2 Put the chipotle paste (or paprika), ketchup, vinegar, Worcestershire sauce and honey in a medium-sized, non-stick pan and mix well. Add the celery, beans and drained sweet potatoes. Heat gently, stirring from time to time, to warm through.

4 Toast the bread on both sides and top with the beans. Serve with rocket, a good grinding of black pepper and a drizzle of olive oil, if you like.

***FOOD.NDTV.COM

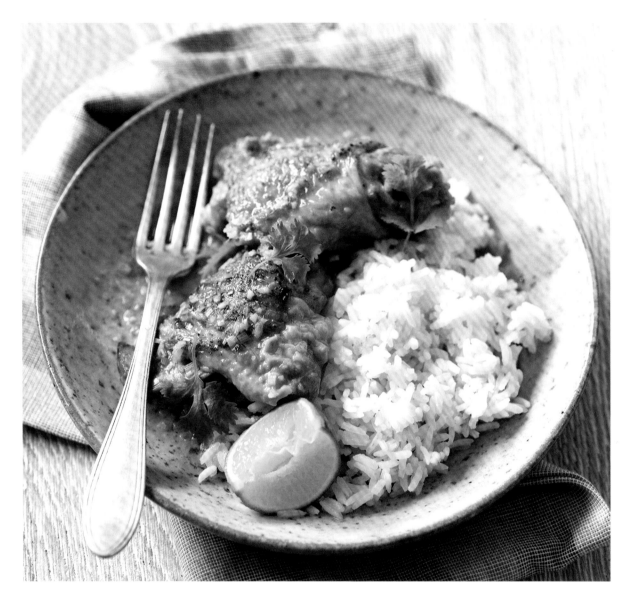

Lemongrass and ginger chicken

Lemongrass has long been used to ward off colds and fevers and it combines well with the garlic and ginger. The chicken provides protein, B vitamins and selenium, which we need for a healthy immune system response.

Serves 4 • 1 hr 10 mins

- **2tbsp fish sauce**
- **1tbsp caster sugar**
- **8 large chicken thighs**
- **3 sticks lemongrass, finely sliced**
- **3 garlic cloves, chopped**
- **6cm (2.5in) fresh root ginger, peeled and chopped**
- **2tbsp groundnut oil**
- **Juice of a lime**
- **2tbsp coriander, chopped**
- **Jasmine rice, to serve**

1 Mix fish sauce and sugar in a large bowl, then add chicken thighs, coating thoroughly in the mixture. Cover the chicken and place in the fridge to marinate for 30 mins.

2 Meanwhile blend sliced lemongrass, chopped garlic and ginger together in a food processor.

3 Heat oil in a large pan. Remove chicken from the marinade, add to the pan and brown well on all sides. Add lemongrass mixture and fry until fragrant.

4 Add marinade and 250ml (9fl oz) water, stir well, cover and simmer over a low heat for 35 mins. Remove lid, add lime juice and chopped coriander, taste and adjust seasoning, then serve with jasmine rice.

Sausage stew with butternut and cannellini beans

Stay full for longer with this healthy dish packed with protein and vitamins.

Serves 4 · 55 mins

- 8 extra-lean sausages (50% reduced fat or as close as you can find)
- 350g (12.3oz) butternut squash, peeled, deseeded and diced
- 1 red onion, cut into wedges
- 400g (14oz) can cherry tomatoes
- 100ml (3.4floz) balsamic vinegar
- 400g (14oz) can cannellini beans
- 2 rosemary sprigs

1 Heat oven to 200°C/390°F/Gas 6. Arrange the sausages, squash and red onion in a large roasting tin and roast in the oven for 30 mins.
2 Turn the sausages and veg over, add the tomatoes and stir in the balsamic vinegar, drained cannellini beans and rosemary sprigs.
3 Cook for 15 mins until everything is piping hot, then serve.

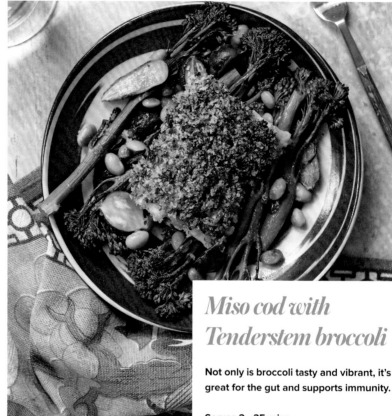

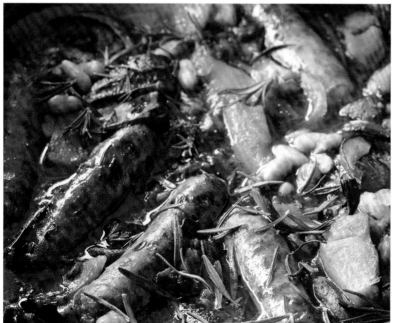

Miso cod with Tenderstem broccoli

Not only is broccoli tasty and vibrant, it's great for the gut and supports immunity.

Serves 2 · 35 mins

- 30g (1oz) panko breadcrumbs
- 1tsp brown rice miso
- 1tbsp olive oil
- Small handful chopped fresh coriander
- 2 pieces of cod loin
- 200g (7oz) Tenderstem broccoli
- 100g (3.5oz) edamame beans
- 8-10 radishes, cut in half
- Miso soup sachet – we used Itsu
- 1tbsp rice wine vinegar
- 1tsp sesame oil
- 1tsp honey
- ½tsp light soy sauce

1 Heat the oven to 200°C/390°F/Gas 6. Mix the breadcrumbs with the miso, oil and coriander. Coat the top of each cod loin with the panko mixture and set aside.
2 Layer the bottom of a deep roasting tin with the broccoli, beans and radishes.
3 Mix the miso soup sachet with 200ml (7fl oz) boiling water, rice wine vinegar, sesame oil, honey and soy sauce. Pour over the veg and roast for 5 mins. Remove from oven and place the cod on top. Bake for a further 20 mins.

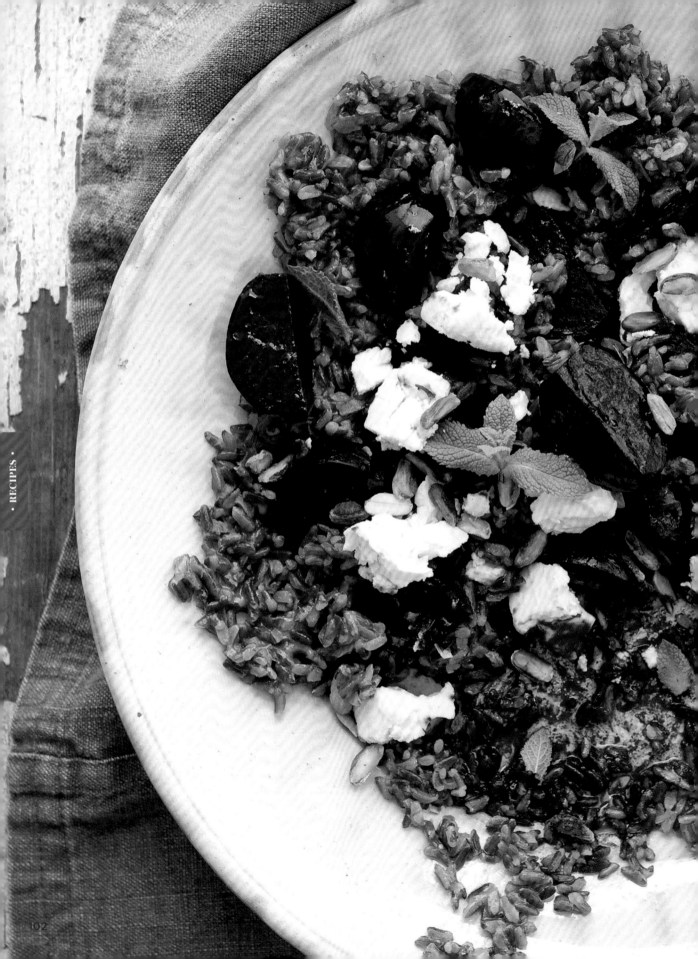

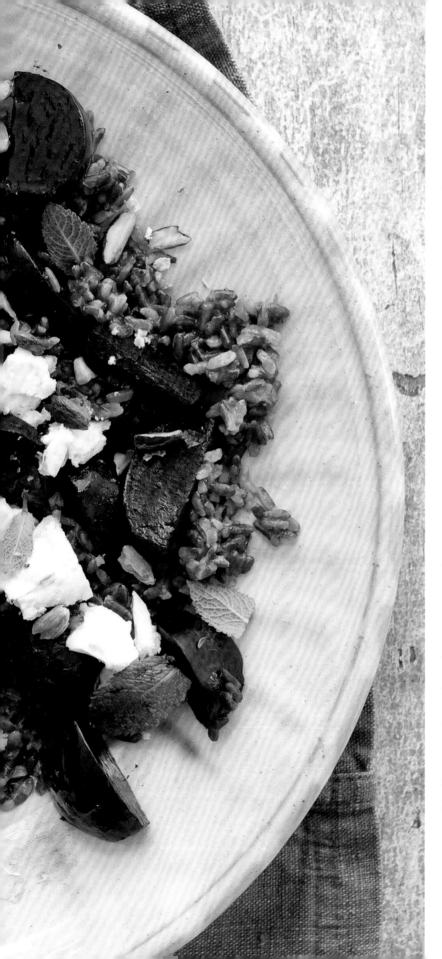

Brown rice and beetroot salad

Beetroot contains nitrates which help dilate blood vessels and bring oxygen-rich blood to the brain. Wholegrains, like brown rice, contain nutrients that are vital for strong brain health.

Serves: 4 • Takes 1 hr 30 mins

- **500g (17.6oz) uncooked beetroot (about 4 or 5 beets)**
- **Juice and grated zest of 1 orange**
- **2tbsp olive oil**
- **150g (5.3oz) brown rice**
- **2tbsp shelled pistachios, roughly chopped**
- **100g (3.5oz) feta, crumbled**
- **Good handful of mint leaves, roughly chopped or left whole if small**

1 Preheat the oven to 180°C/355°F/Gas 4. Trim the beetroot, leaving a little bit of stalk on each one, then put them in a roasting tin. Cover loosely with foil and bake for about 1 hr 30 mins in the oven, depending on their size, until they are tender. While the beetroot are still warm, peel, quarter and slice them, then put in a mixing bowl with the orange juice and zest, and the oil.
2 Meanwhile, add the rice to a pan of boiling water and simmer for 30 mins. Drain and leave to cool, then add to the bowl of beetroot.
3 Stir in the pistachios, feta and mint. Season well, then gently mix the salad. Transfer to a dish to serve.

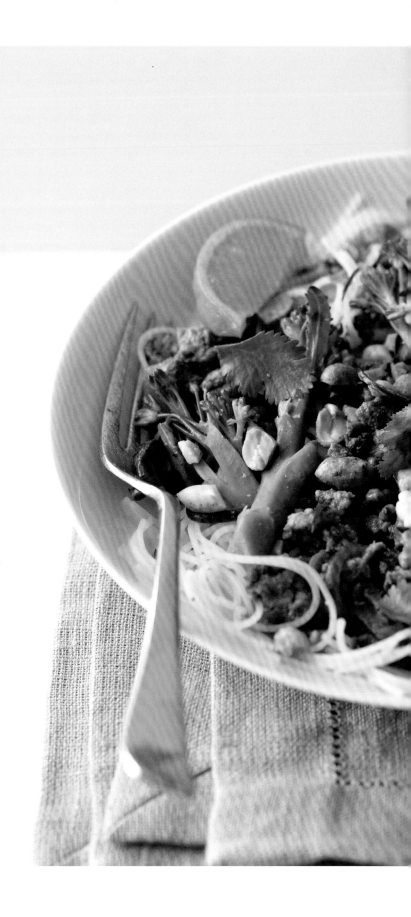

Thai-style stir-fried mince with broccoli and rice noodles

Broccoli is often called the ultimate brain food – it can help preserve memory, improve your ability to learn and promote brain healing.

Serves 2 · Takes 20 mins

- 200g (7oz) rice vermicelli noodles
- 2tbsp oil
- 1 red onion, sliced
- 2 cloves garlic, chopped
- 2 red chillies, deseeded and finely sliced
- 200g (7oz) lean minced beef
- 100g (3.5oz) Tenderstem broccoli, halved lengthways
- 2tbsp fish sauce
- 1tbsp light soy sauce
- 1tsp sugar
- 1tsp sesame oil
- Small handful of dry roasted peanuts
- Small handful of coriander leaves
- 1 lime cut into wedges

1 Put the noodles in a bowl, pour over some boiling water, cover and leave for 8 mins, until softened.
2 Meanwhile, heat the oil in a wok and fry the onion, garlic and chilli for 2 mins. Add the mince, breaking up the clumps, and stir-fry over a high heat for 8 mins.
3 Stir in the broccoli, fish sauce, soy sauce and sugar and cook for 4 mins.
4 Drain the noodles, then toss them together with the sesame oil. Combine the noodles and mince, and serve in bowls topped with peanuts, coriander leaves and a lime wedge.

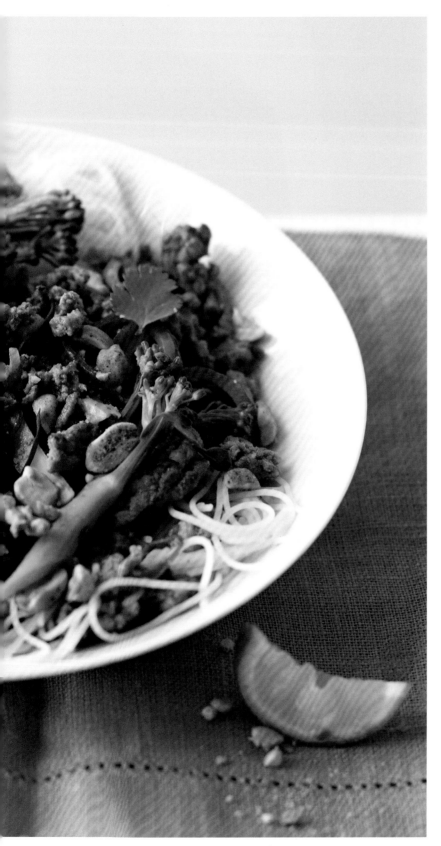

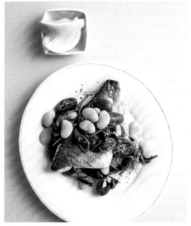

Sea bass with spinach, tomatoes and butter beans

Sea bass, spinach and tomatoes all contain substances that help increase your brain power and concentration, so give this speedy recipe a try if your brain needs a boost.

Serves 1 • Takes 15 mins

- **Frylight Extra Virgin Olive Oil Spray**
- **125g (4.4oz) sea bass fillet**
- **5 cherry tomatoes, halved**
- **1 garlic clove, crushed**
- **125g (4.4oz) baby spinach leaves**
- **200g (7oz) can butter beans, drained**
- **2 lemon wedges**

1 Heat a non-stick frying pan with a couple of squirts of the olive oil spray.
2 Season the fish and sear it skin side down, cooking for 3 mins or until crisp. Turn the fish over, push to one side and cook for a couple more mins.
3 Add the tomatoes, garlic, spinach and butter beans and cook for a couple of mins to wilt the spinach. Remove the fish and check the butter beans are warmed through. Serve the fish and veg together.

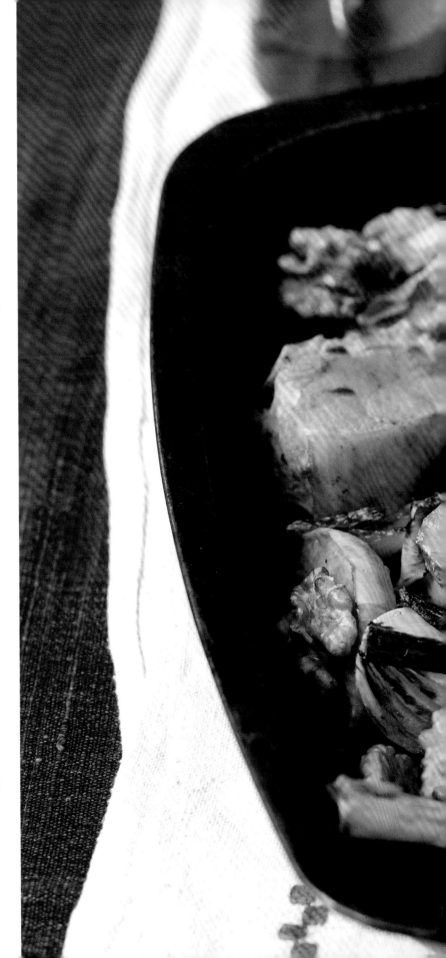

Lamb with squash, walnuts and sage

'Red meats are rich in zinc, essential to the immune system,' explains nutritionist Kim Pearson. Zinc helps heal wounds and fight infections so, if you're a meat-eater, choose red meat like beef, pork and lamb. 'It's vital for the primary immunity gland, the thymus, and required for white blood cell production,' says Shabir Daya, pharmacist and co-founder of victoriahealth.com. Eat red meat in moderation – the NHS recommends 70g daily. Lentils, chickpeas and chia seeds are also rich zinc sources.

Serves 4 · Cook 50 mins

- 2 onions, peeled, cut into wedges
- 1 butternut squash, peeled, deseeded and cut into wedges
- 3tbsp olive oil
- 400g (14.1oz) French-trimmed rack of lamb
- 90g (3.2oz) walnut halves
- Handful of fresh sage
- 2tbsp balsamic or sherry vinegar

1 Preheat oven to 200°C/400°F/Gas 6. In a tin, roast onions and squash, seasoned and drizzled with oil, for 30 mins. Meanwhile, brown lamb in a hot pan for 2 mins on each side, add to veg in tin, and sprinkle with nuts and sage. Cook for 15-20 mins.
2 Take lamb out, wrap in foil and leave to rest. Stir veg well and cook for 10 mins more. Cut the lamb into chops, return them to the tin and spoon over the vinegar to serve.

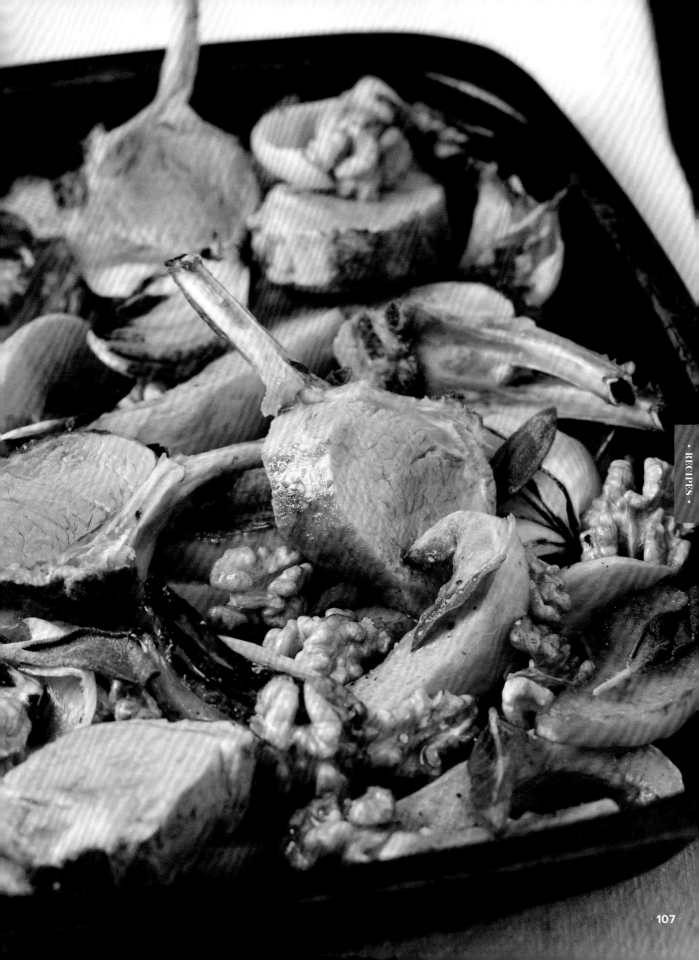

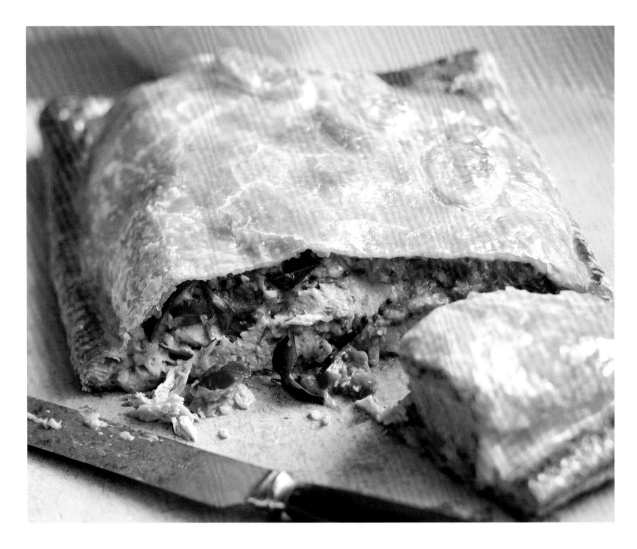

Kerala curried salmon slice

Salmon is rich in omega-3. 'Omega-3 fats help us fight infections such as colds and flu,' says nutritionist Babi Chana. 'Disease-producing "bugs" attack us when immune function is poor, so up omega-3 fats to safeguard against coughs and colds.'

Serves 8 • Cook 1 hr

- 2 x 375g (13.2oz) sheets ready-rolled puff pastry
- 850g (30oz) piece of salmon fillet
- 1 onion, quartered
- 2 garlic cloves, peeled
- 1 red chilli, deseeded
- 50g (1.8oz) fresh coconut pieces
- 1tbsp sunflower oil
- ½tsp ground black pepper
- 1tsp black mustard seeds
- 6-12 curry leaves
- 1tsp ground turmeric
- 227g (8oz) can chopped tomatoes
- 150ml (5floz) coconut milk
- 1½tbsp polenta
- 1 egg, beaten

1 Heat oven to 200°C/400°F/Gas 6. Unroll one sheet of pastry on a baking tray and trim to 3cm (1.2in) larger all round than salmon. Prick pastry with a fork, cover with another baking tray and bake for 15 mins. Remove top baking tray and bake for 5 mins until golden.

2 Meanwhile whizz onion, garlic, chilli and coconut in a food processor to make a paste. Heat oil in a pan, add paste and cook for a few mins. Add pepper, mustard seeds and curry leaves, cook for 1 min, then add the turmeric, tomatoes and coconut milk. Simmer for 20 mins, stirring, until thickened. Cool slightly.

3 Sprinkle polenta over the cooked pastry, place salmon on top, then spoon over the curry. Brush pastry edges with beaten egg, then lay the remaining pastry sheet on top. Trim off excess and press edges with a fork to seal. Brush with beaten egg and bake for 30 mins.

Lentil, sausage and fennel salad

Get into the habit of using a good extra virgin olive oil for dressings, not just for the extra flavour but the extra health benefits.

Serves 4 • Ready in 1 hr

- 3 red onions, peeled, halved and cut into wedges
- 6 thyme sprigs, plus 1tsp leaves
- 6 lean pork or chicken sausages
- 1½tbsp olive oil
- 200g (7oz) puy lentils
- 2 fennel bulbs, trimmed and finely sliced

For the dressing:
- 1tsp Dijon mustard
- 4tbsp extra virgin olive oil
- 2tbsp balsamic vinegar
- 1tbsp mild-flavoured honey

1 Heat the oven to 190°C/375°F/Gas 5. Lay the onions and thyme in a single layer in a roasting tin and arrange the sausages on top. Drizzle with the oil and roast for around 35 mins, until the sausages are golden brown and the onions are soft.

2 Meanwhile, put the lentils in a saucepan and cover with plenty of cold water. Bring to the boil, then reduce the heat to a simmer, partially cover the pan and cook for 20 mins. The lentils should be soft, but still retain their shape. Drain and transfer to a large bowl.

3 Whisk all the dressing ingredients together with 1tbsp of warm water and season well. Stir half the dressing into the lentils and check the seasoning. Thickly slice the sausages and combine with the lentils, onions, extra thyme and fennel. Serve with the remaining dressing spooned over.

HEALTH TIP
Extra virgin olive oil, a key ingredient of the healthy Mediterranean diet, has been proven to destroy cancer cells

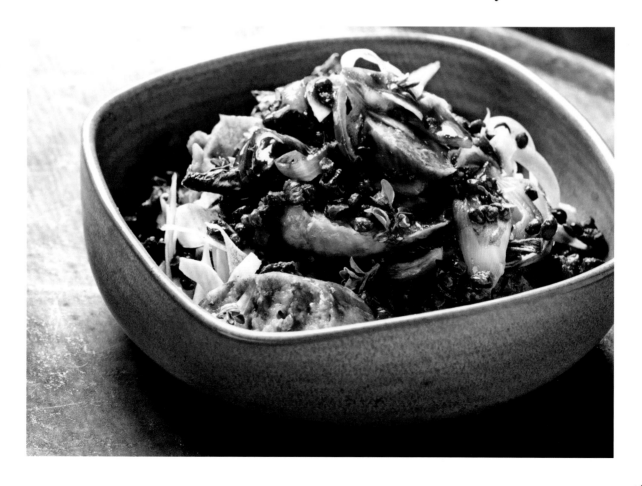

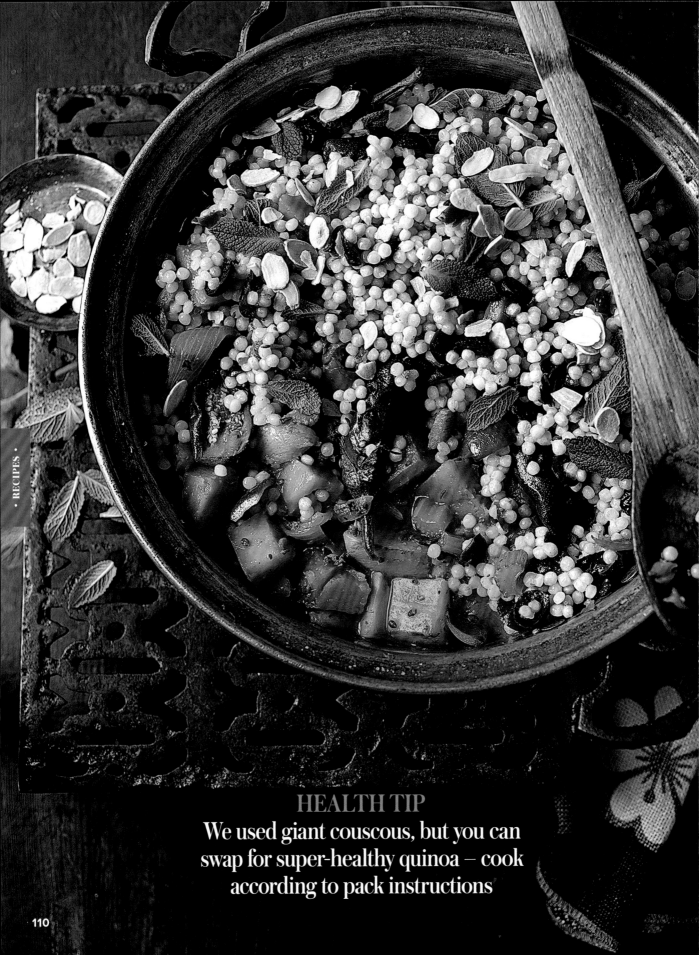

HEALTH TIP
We used giant couscous, but you can
swap for super-healthy quinoa – cook
according to pack instructions

Persian-style vegetable casserole

Aromatic spices transform humble vegetables into a jewelled feast.

Serves 6 • Ready in 1 hr 15 mins

- 200g (7oz) giant couscous
- 75g (2.6oz) Craisins/dried cranberries
- 1 small celeriac, peeled and cut into 2cm (0.8in) chunks
- 3tbsp sunflower oil
- 1 large carrot, cut into small chunks
- 2 red onions, roughly chopped
- 2 sticks of celery, sliced 1cm (0.4in) thick
- 2tbsp coriander seeds, crushed
- 2tsp cumin seeds, crushed
- ½tsp chilli flakes
- 100g (3.5oz) dried apricots, quartered
- Pinch of saffron (about third of a 0.4g pack), soaked in 750ml (25fl oz) boiling water
- 1tbsp low-salt vegetable stock powder
- 200g (7oz) baby aubergines, halved
- 1 small butternut squash, peeled and cut into 2.5cm (1in) chunks
- Juice of 1 lemon
- Small bunch of mint, leaves only
- 30g (1oz) toasted flaked almonds

1 Mix the couscous and Craisins with 750ml (25fl oz) boiling water, cover, leave for 20 mins. Drain.
2 In a big pan, fry the celeriac in half the oil for 5 mins, until golden. Transfer to a bowl. Fry the carrot, onion and celery in remaining oil for 5 mins, stirring. Add the spices and apricots and cook for 2 mins. Mix the saffron water with the stock powder and add to pan. Bring to a boil, cover and simmer for 10 mins.
3 Add the aubergine and squash, stir, cover and cook for 10 mins. Stir in the lemon juice, season, then scatter the couscous over. Heat gently for 5 mins, until piping hot. Serve scattered with mint and almonds.

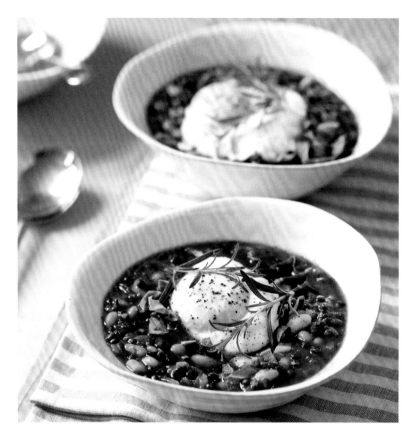

Super bean and lentil soup

A hearty bowl that delivers several of your 5-a-day. This serves four generously, but any leftovers make a perfect lunch.

Serves 4-6 • Ready in 40 mins

- 1tbsp oil
- 2 onions, finely chopped
- 1 stick celery, finely chopped
- 2 garlic cloves, crushed
- 1l (1.7pt) low-salt vegetable stock
- 400g (14oz) can chopped tomatoes
- 3 sprigs rosemary, finely chopped
- 400g (14oz) can cannellini beans, drained and rinsed
- 200g (7oz) can flageolet beans, drained and rinsed
- 250g (8.8oz) pack cooked puy lentils
- 4 free-range eggs
- 100g (3.5oz) spring greens or sprout tops, shredded
- Fresh rosemary sprigs, to serve (optional)

1 Heat the oil in a large pan and sweat the onions and celery for 10 mins. Add the garlic and cook for a couple of mins then add the stock, tomatoes and rosemary. Bring to the boil then simmer for 10 mins.
2 Add the beans. Microwave the lentils for a few mins then add them, too. Keep the soup simmering while you poach the eggs.
3 Bring a sauté pan of water to the boil then turn it down to a very low simmer. Break the eggs one by one into a ramekin and gently tip into the water. Put on the lid and cook for 3 mins. Add the greens to the soup and top each bowl with a poached egg and some rosemary, if liked.

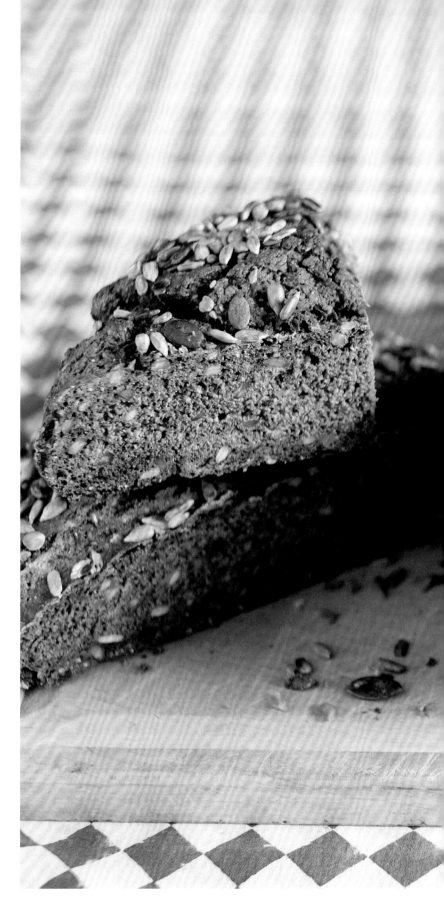

Soda bread

Cuts into 10 slices • Ready in 1 hr

- **200g (7oz) rye flour**
- **100g (3.5oz) plain white flour**
- **1½tsp bicarbonate of soda**
- **1½tsp sea salt**
- **3tbsp mixed seeds, plus extra for sprinkling**
- **1tbsp black treacle**
- **284ml (9.6fl oz) carton buttermilk**
- **Oil, for greasing**
- **Milk, for brushing**

1 Heat the oven to 200°C/400°F/Gas 6. Mix together the rye and plain white flours with the bicarbonate of soda, sea salt and mixed seeds.
2 Make a well in the centre, and add the treacle and the carton of buttermilk. Mix well then shape into a round. Place on an oiled baking sheet. Put a cross right through (use a long wooden spoon handle), brush with a little milk and scatter more seeds over the top. Bake for 45 mins, or until the base sounds hollow when tapped.

HEALTH TIP
Butternut squash is rich in antioxidants and vitamins that can reduce the risk of certain cancers

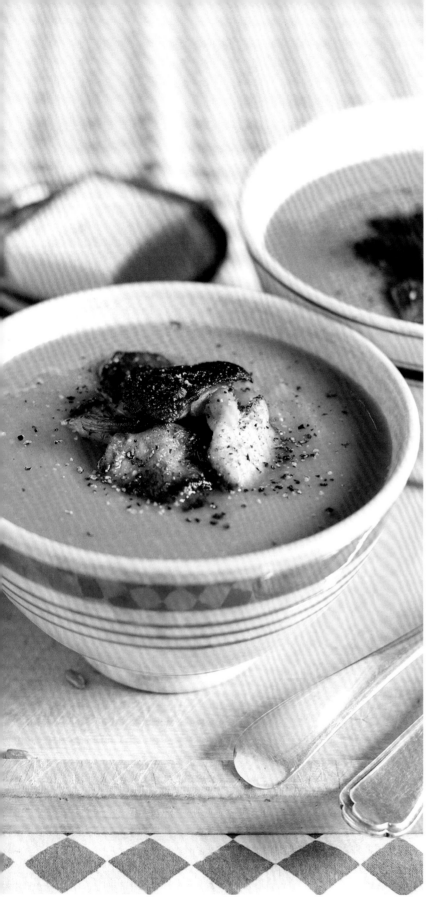

Butternut squash soup with shiitake mushrooms

This nourishing soup is a nutritious alternative to a lunchtime sandwich. Eat the bread on the day it is made, or freeze.

Serves 6 • Ready in 50 mins

- **1tbsp olive oil**
- **1 medium onion, roughly chopped**
- **3 garlic cloves, crushed**
- **1tsp cayenne pepper**
- **1tsp ground cinnamon**
- **3 sprigs thyme**
- **1.8kg (4lb) butternut squash, peeled, deseeded and roughly chopped**
- **700ml (23.6fl oz) veg or chicken stock**
- **100ml (3.4fl oz) milk**
- **125g (4.4oz) shiitake mushrooms**

1 Heat half the oil in a large saucepan over a medium heat. Cook the onion for 3 or 4 mins, or until just starting to brown. Add the garlic, cayenne pepper, cinnamon and thyme, and cook for another 1 or 2 mins, stirring often.

2 Add the squash and stock, bring to the boil then leave to simmer for 20 to 25 mins, or until the squash is tender. Pour in the milk and season well, remove from the heat and blend until smooth. Keep warm until ready to serve.

3 Heat the remaining oil in a small, heavy-based frying pan to medium high. Sauté the mushrooms for 3 or 4 mins, or until crispy. Divide the mushrooms between each bowl of soup as a topping.

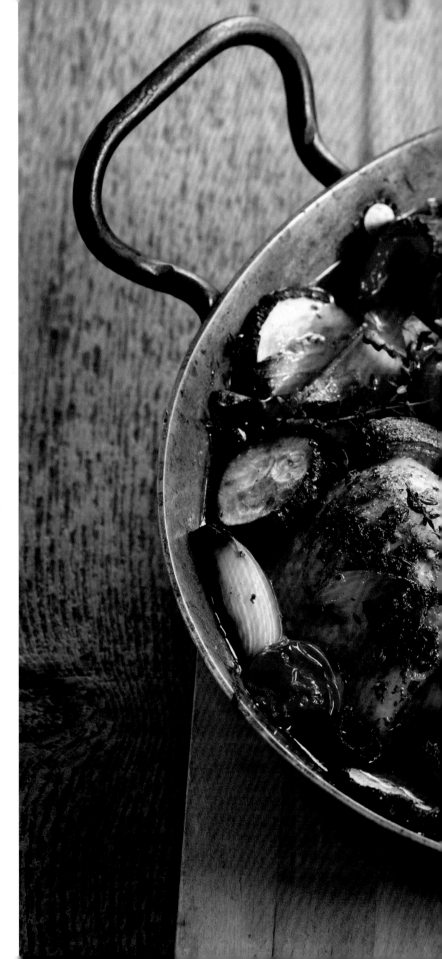

Zesty Mediterranean chicken

A fuss-free midweek meal that is packed with fibre-rich vegetables.

Serves 4 • Ready in 40 mins

- **6 chicken thighs**
- **2tsp chicken seasoning**
- **400g (14oz) pack ready-to-roast Mediterranean vegetables (including onions, courgettes, peppers and cherry tomatoes)**
- **2 garlic cloves, crushed**
- **Juice of 2 lemons**
- **2tbsp olive oil**
- **Thyme sprigs, to serve (optional)**
- **Extra or salad or vegetables, to serve**

1 Heat the oven to 200°C/400°F/Gas 6. Put the chicken thighs in a large roasting tin and season with freshly ground black pepper and the chicken seasoning.
2 Add the Mediterranean vegetables and crushed garlic and pour over the lemon juice and olive oil.
3 Roast in the oven for 30-35 mins until the chicken is golden and cooked through and the vegetables are tender. Scatter with thyme sprigs, to serve.

HEALTH TIP
Add a can of drained and rinsed cannellini beans to the dish just before the end of cooking for an extra fibre and 5-a-day boost

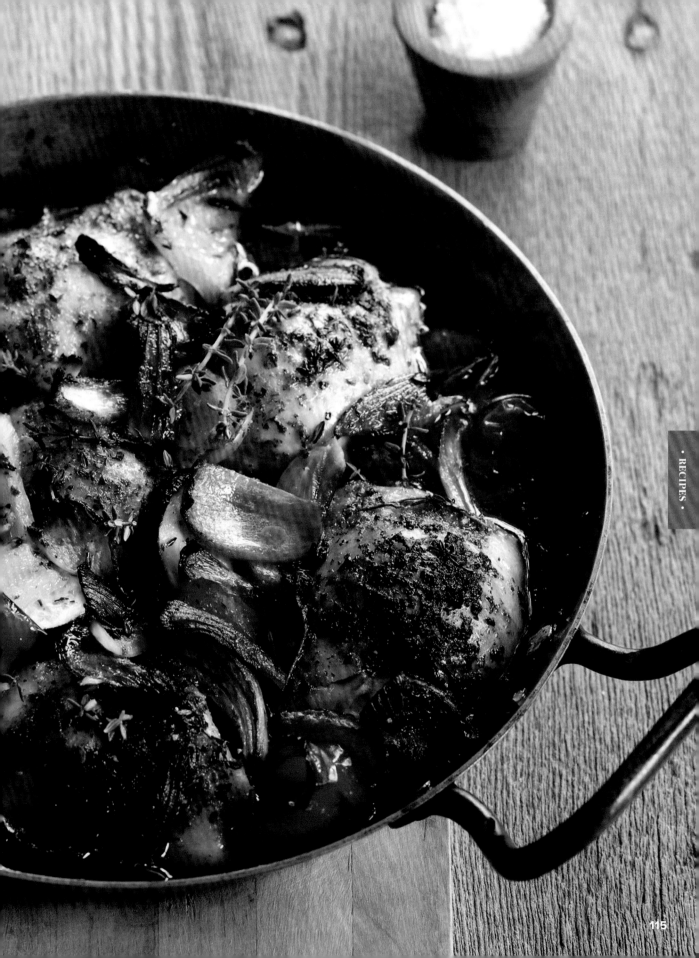

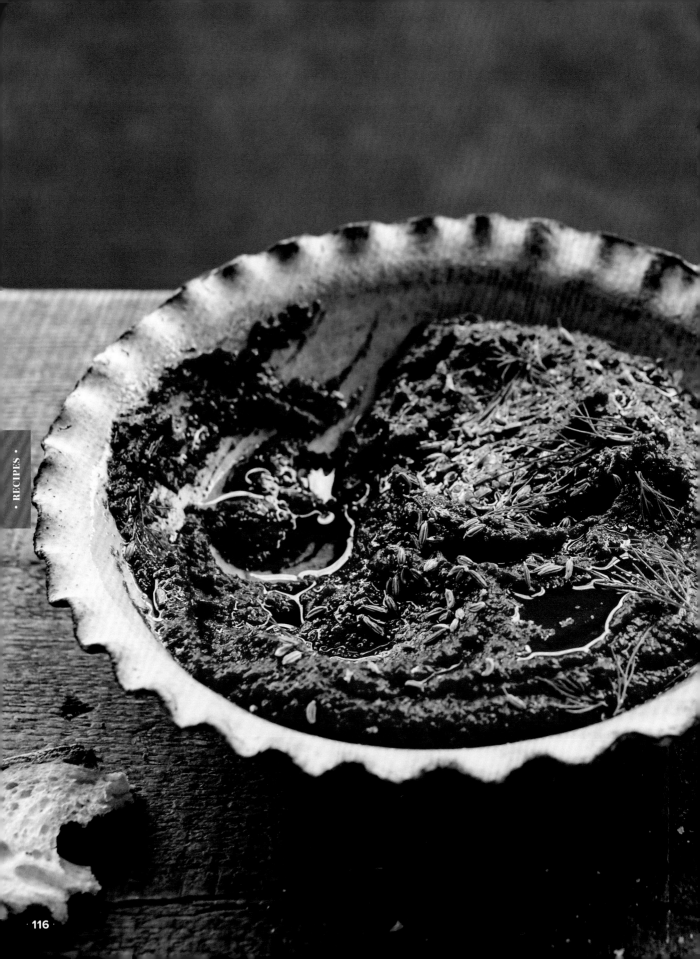

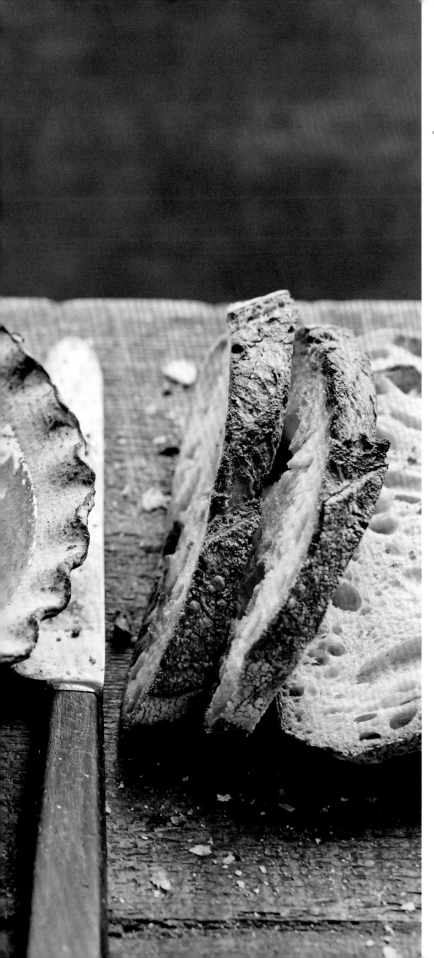

Beetroot and fennel houmous

Beetroot is a bright choice in all ways – for colour, flavour and with nitrates for lowering blood pressure.

Serve 4 • Ready in 50 mins

- 4 small beetroot
- 1 small fennel bulb, trimmed and tops reserved for garnish olive oil
- 1 tin organic chickpeas, drained and rinsed
- 1 fat garlic clove, peeled and crushed
- 1tsp fennel seeds, plus extra to garnish
- 1tbsp tahini
- Generous squeeze of lemon juice
- 100ml (3.4floz) extra virgin olive oil

1 Heat the oven to 200°C/400°F/Gas 6. Wrap each beetroot individually in foil and put in a roasting tin. Slice the fennel and toss with a little oil in a separate small roasting tin, then season with freshly ground black pepper.
2 Put both tins in the oven and roast for 40 mins, until the fennel is softened and the beetroot is tender to the tip of a knife.
3 Once the beetroot are cool, peel them and put into a food processor with the roasted fennel, chickpeas, garlic, fennel seeds, tahini and lemon juice. Blitz to form a smooth paste, drizzling in the extra virgin olive oil as you go. Loosen with a little cold water if it is too thick. Garnish with fennel tops and fennel seeds.

HEALTH TIP
Roasting beetroot maximises the nitrate benefits. Nitrates are water-soluble, so are lost when you boil them

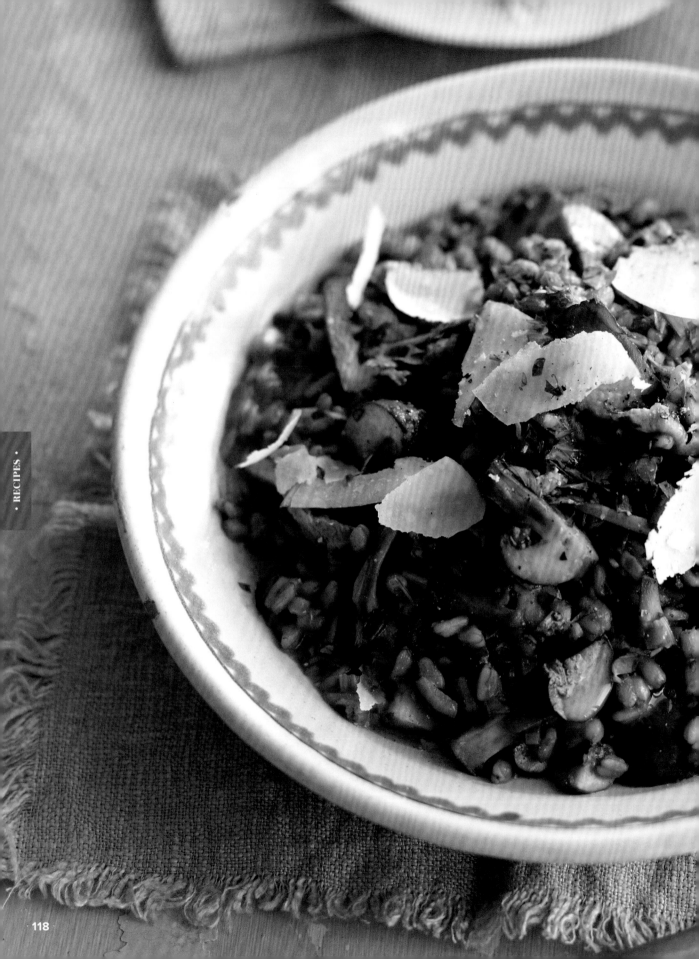

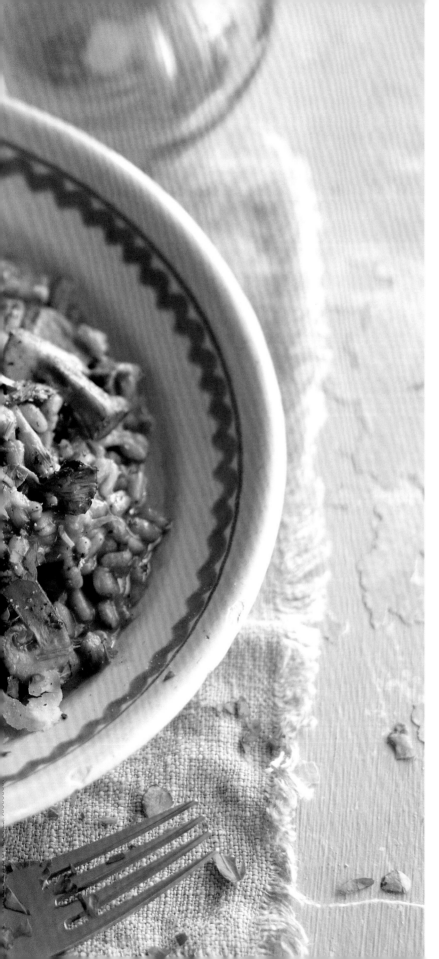

Mixed mushrooms and spelt

Spelt is an ancient grain that is high in fibre and nutrients linked to a reduced risk of heart disease.

Serves 6 • Ready in 40 mins

- **2tbsp olive oil, plus extra**
- **1 large onion, chopped**
- **1 stick celery, chopped**
- **1 carrot peeled and chopped**
- **2 garlic cloves**
- **200g (7oz) chestnut mushrooms, chopped**
- **350g (12.3oz) spelt**
- **200ml (6.7fl oz) red wine**
- **1.2l (40fl oz) hot beef stock**
- **100g (3.5oz) pack wild mushrooms**
- **Parmesan shavings and chopped parsley, to garnish**

1 Heat the oil and cook the onion, celery, carrot and garlic for 10 mins. Add the chestnut mushrooms and cook for a further 2 mins. Stir in the spelt, then add the wine. Cook until the wine has absorbed. Add the stock and simmer for 25 mins, or until the spelt is tender.
2 Fry the wild mushrooms in a little oil and add to the spelt mixture, along with the Parmesan shavings and the fresh parsley.

HEALTH TIP
Onions contain quercetin that can also help reduce blood pressure

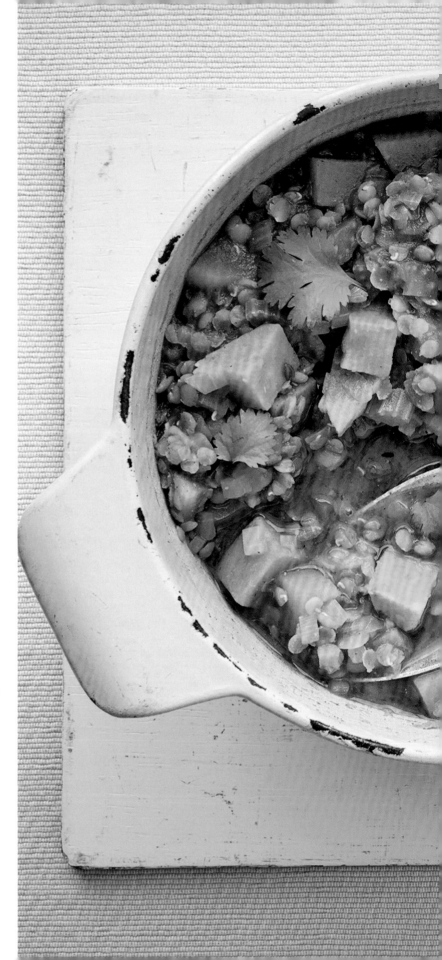

HEALTH TIP
Eating garlic regularly can help lower blood pressure and cholesterol

Sweet potato, squash and lentil casserole

A delicious, subtly spiced low-fat but hearty meat-free dinner.

Serves 4 • Ready in 45 mins

- **1tbsp olive oil**
- **2 celery sticks, thinly sliced**
- **1 onion, chopped**
- **2 garlic cloves, roughly chopped**
- **350g (12.3oz) mix of sweet potato and butternut squash, cut into bite-sized pieces**
- **1 Granny Smith apple, peeled and chopped**
- **1tbsp medium curry powder**
- **100g (3.5oz) red lentils, rinsed**
- **1 vegetable stock cube**
- **1tbsp tomato purée**
- **1tbsp mango chutney**
- **Fresh coriander leaves, to garnish**

1 Heat the oil in a large pan and cook the celery, onion and garlic for 8-10 mins, until beginning to soften.
2 Add the sweet potato and butternut squash to the pan along with the apple, curry powder and lentils. Cook, stirring, for a further 2 mins. Add 650ml (22fl oz) hot water to the pan with the stock cube, tomato purée and mango chutney. Bring to the boil, then reduce the heat and simmer gently for around 25 mins, until the vegetables and lentils are tender. Serve ladled into deep bowls, garnished with coriander leaves.

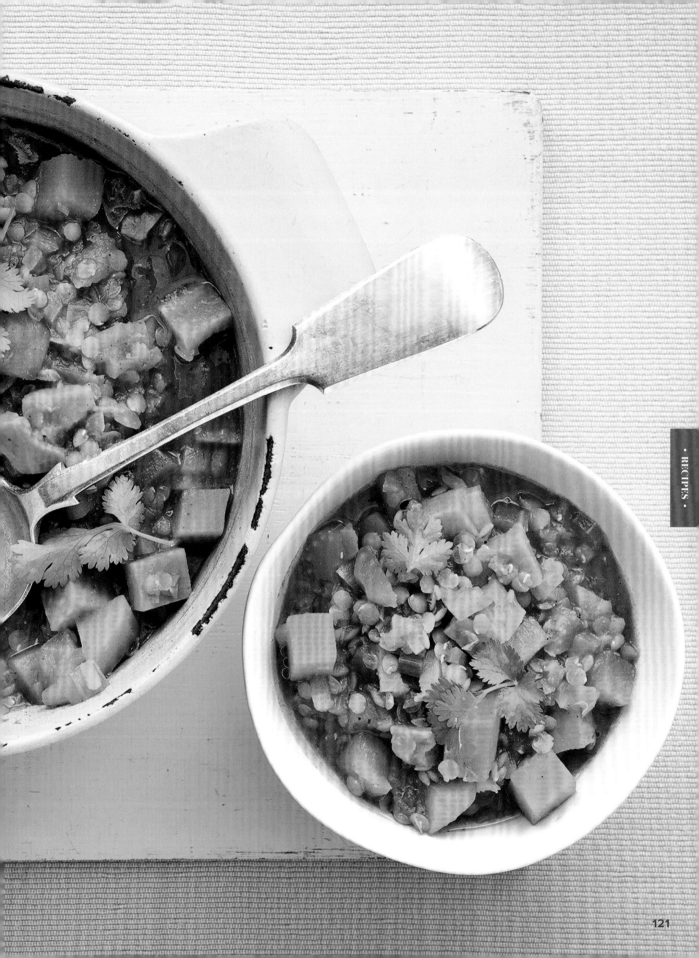

Gado gado

Tofu is good for those on dairy-free diets.

Serves 6 • Ready in 40 mins

- **500g (17.5oz) sweet potatoes, cubed**
- **1 courgette, cubed**
- **1 red pepper, deseeded and chopped**
- **1 cauliflower, cut into florets**
- **2 garlic cloves, crushed**
- **4tbsp olive oil**
- **200g (7oz) green beans**
- **200g (7oz) marinated tofu**
- **1 small bunch coriander, chopped**
- **60g (2.1oz) salted peanuts, chopped**
- **Lime wedges, to serve**

For the peanut dressing:
- **1tbsp sunflower oil**
- **1 red onion, chopped**
- **4 garlic cloves, chopped**
- **1 red chilli, deseeded and chopped**
- **1tsp tamari or soy sauce**
- **4 lime leaves, chopped**
- **250ml (8.4floz) coconut cream**
- **200g (7oz) jar crunchy peanut butter**

1 Heat the oven to 200°C/400°F/Gas 6. Spread the sweet potatoes, courgette and red pepper out in a roasting tin. Spread the cauliflower out in another tin. Sprinkle the garlic over the veg and drizzle with oil. Roast for 25 mins, then cool.

2 To make the peanut dressing, heat the oil in a pan and fry the red onion for a few mins, to soften. Add the garlic and chilli. Cook for 1 min, then add the rest of the dressing ingredients and 150ml (5fl oz) boiling water. Stir until smooth. Cool.

3 Cook the green beans with 2tbsp water on High in the microwave for 3 mins. Drain and rinse under cold water.

4 Divide the dressing between 6 bowls. Spoon on the cooled roasted veg, beans and tofu. Sprinkle with coriander and peanuts. Serve with lime wedges.

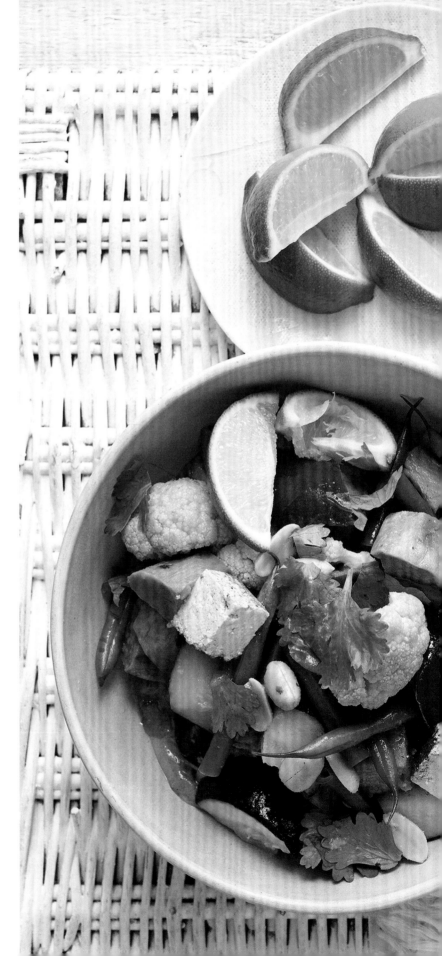

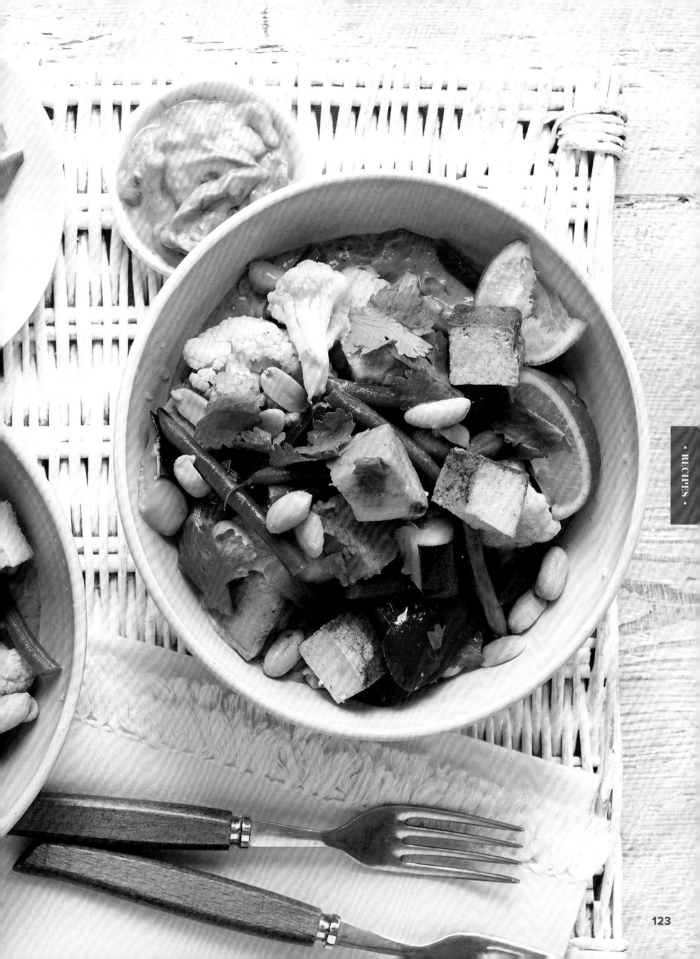

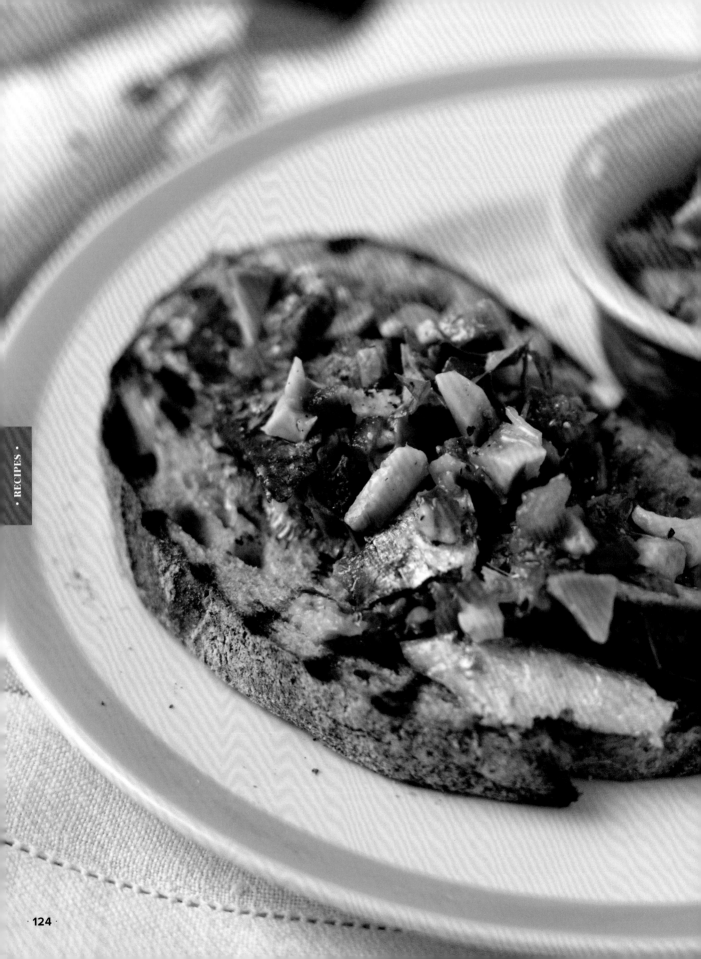

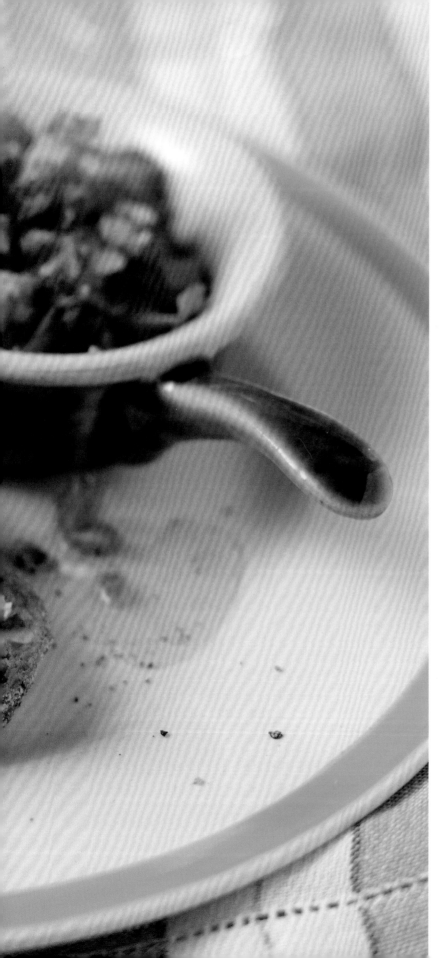

Sardines with avocado salsa

This fish, eaten bones and all, is an excellent source of calcium.

Serves 2 • Ready in 15 mins

- **100g (3.5oz) can sardines in oil**
- **4 slices sourdough bread**

For the salsa:
- **1 ripe avocado**
- **½ small red onion, finely chopped**
- **4 tomatoes, deseeded and chopped**
- **½ red chilli, deseeded and chopped**
- **Juice ½ lime**
- **1tbsp fresh coriander, chopped**

1 Make the salsa first, peel the avocado and remove the stone. Dice the flesh and place in a bowl with the red onion, tomatoes, red chilli, lime juice and coriander. Season to taste.
2 Drain the sardines and break them up a little using a fork. Toast the sourdough bread, then place the sardines on top and serve topped with the salsa.

HEALTH TIP
A can of sardines contributes around 6mcg vitamin D to an adult's daily requirement of 15-20mcg

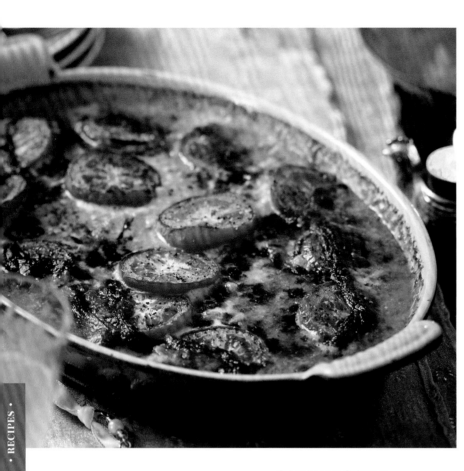

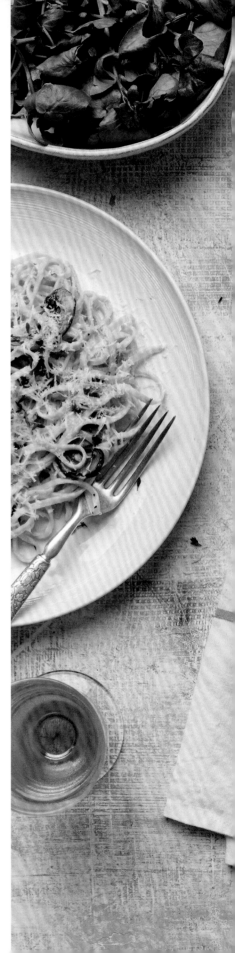

Smoked haddock rarebit

Adding beer and mustard to this cheesy bake gives it a tangy, spicy kick.

Serves 6 • Ready in 20 mins

- 750g (26.4oz) smoked haddock fillets
- 250ml (8.4floz) semi-skimmed milk
- 500g (17.5oz) mature Cheddar cheese, grated
- 3tsp Worcestershire sauce
- 3tsp dried mustard powder
- 2tbsp beer or Guinness
- 4 large tomatoes, sliced

1 Put the haddock and milk in a pan and bring to a boil, then reduce to a simmer for 4-5 mins, until the haddock is cooked. Remove the haddock, take off any skin and set aside. When cool enough to handle, pull into large chunks.

2 Mix together the grated cheese, Worcestershire sauce, mustard powder and beer or Guinness.

3 Put the haddock into a large baking dish and top with the cheesy rarebit mix and sliced tomatoes. Cook under a hot grill for 10-15 mins or until browned and bubbling.

HEALTH TIP Milk and cheese are some of the best and most readily available sources of bone-friendly calcium

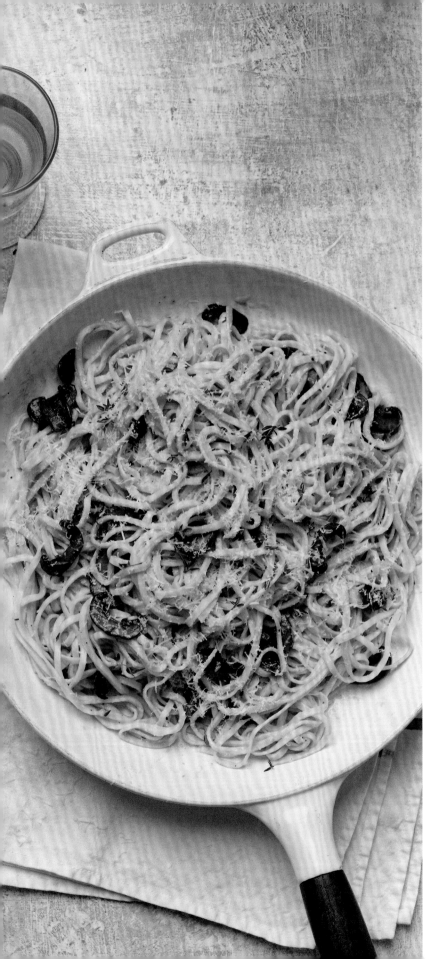

Veggie carbonara

A deliciously rich and satisfying dish.

Serves 4 • Ready in 25 mins

- 200g (7oz) vitamin-D enriched chestnut mushrooms
- 1 garlic clove
- 2tbsp olive oil
- 3 medium eggs and 2 egg yolks
- 45g (1.5oz) vegetarian smoked cheese, finely grated
- 45g (1.5oz) vegetarian Pecorino, finely grated, plus extra to serve
- 300g (10.5oz) fresh tagliatelle
- Fresh thyme, to serve

1 Dry-fry the mushrooms in a pan for 7-8 mins, to release all their water. Crush the garlic with the back of your hand. Add to the pan with the oil and a generous amount of freshly ground black pepper. Allow the garlic to fry and flavour the oil for 2-3 mins before discarding.
2 In a bowl, whisk the eggs, egg yolks and the cheeses together, then set aside. The egg-and-cheese mix may curdle when combined, but don't worry about it.
3 Meanwhile, in a pan of boiling salted water, cook the pasta for 2 mins until al dente. Reserving some of the liquid, drain the pasta, then add it to the pan and toss to coat in the oil and mushrooms.
4 Working quickly, pour in the egg-and-cheese mixture and toss together, adding a little of the reserved pasta water. Toss until the mixture emulsifies and becomes creamy and silky. Grate over more Pecorino and sprinkle with thyme.

HEALTH TIP
Very few foods contain vitamin D, but egg yolks and mushrooms are both good ways to get it

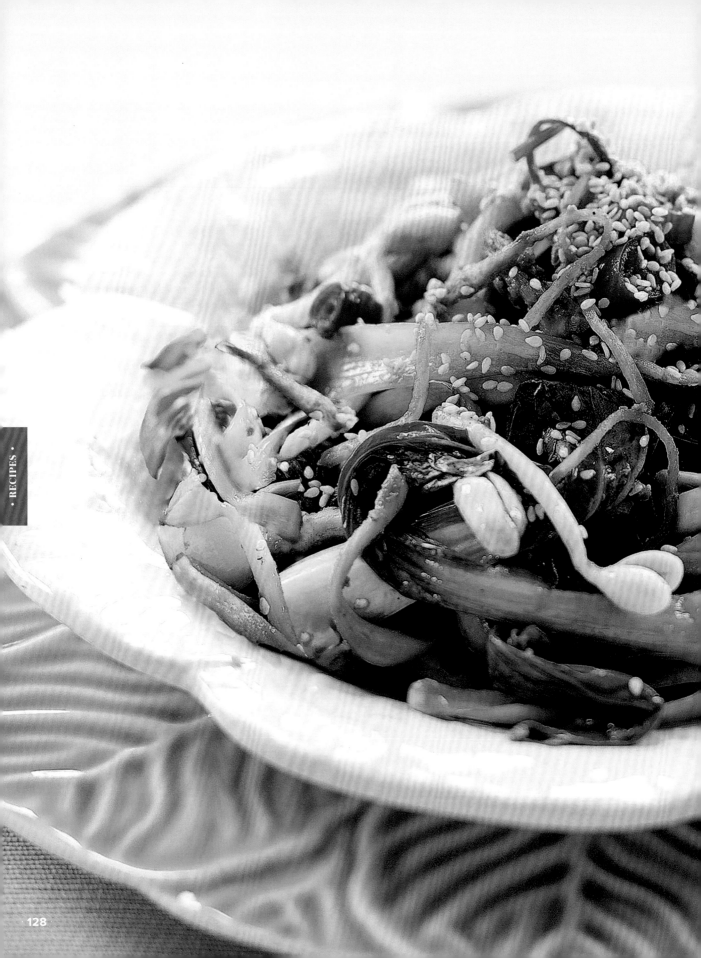

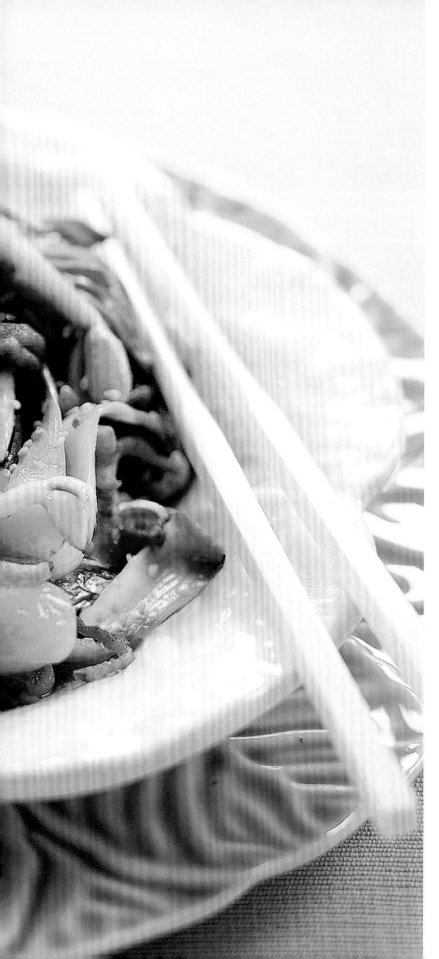

Japanese-style veggie stir-fry

This colour bowl will help to calm things down.

Serves 4 • Ready in 15 mins

- **1tbsp sunflower oil**
- **2tbsp frozen chopped shallots**
- **2 garlic cloves, crushed**
- **3cm (1.2in) piece fresh ginger, chopped**
- **2 packs baby pak choi, cut in half**
- **250g (8.8oz) peanut shoots or bean sprouts**
- **4tbsp Japanese soy sauce**
- **4tbsp rice wine**
- **2tbsp rice vinegar**
- **1tbsp sesame oil**
- **2x300g (10.6oz) packs fresh egg noodles**
- **2tbsp sesame seeds**
- **Pickled ginger (optional)**
- **Juice of ½ a lime**

1 Heat the sunflower oil in a large wok, add the shallots, garlic and ginger and cook for 2 mins. Add the pak choi and stir-fry until it starts to wilt. Add the peanut shoots and stir.

2 Mix together the soy sauce, rice wine, rice vinegar and sesame oil and pour into the wok. Add the noodles and sesame seeds and mix well. Serve sprinkled with the pickled ginger, if using, and a squeeze of lime juice.

HEALTH TIP
Sesame seeds are a source of phytoestrogens that can raise falling oestrogen levels

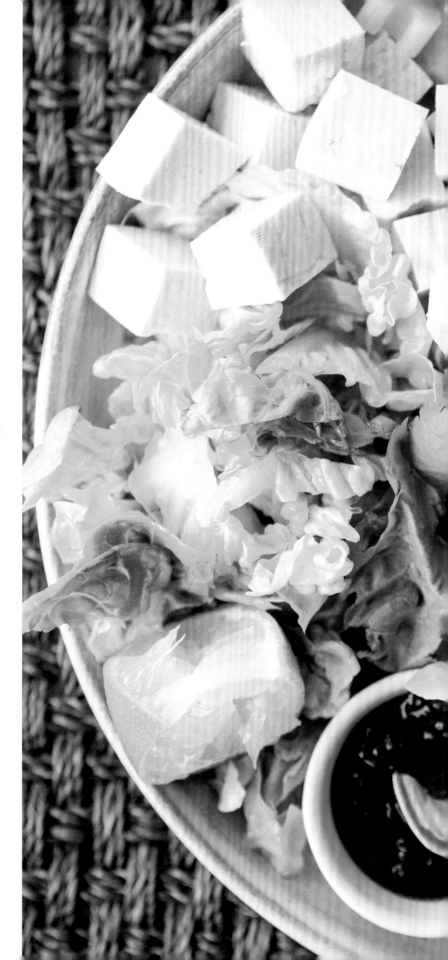

Smoked tofu taco bowl with chilli dressing

This is a good take-to-work lunch – just keep the dressing on the side.

Serves 1 • Ready in 10 mins

- 75g (2.6oz) Little Gem lettuce leaves, shredded
- 60g (2.1oz) smoked tofu
- 1 trimmed salad onion, thinly sliced
- 5 baby plum tomatoes, quartered
- Trimmed celery stick, sliced
- 1tbsp jalapeño pepper slices, drained
- Cucumber, cut in ribbons
- 1tbsp lime juice
- 1tsp sweet chilli jelly
- Handful of coriander leaves

1 Arrange the lettuce, tofu, salad onions, tomatoes, celery, jalapeño and cucumber in a bowl, keeping each one as a separate section.
2 Whisk the lime juice into the sweet chilli jelly and drizzle over the taco bowl. Scatter with coriander leaves.

HEALTH TIP
Celery has a diuretic effect that helps eliminate excess body fluid

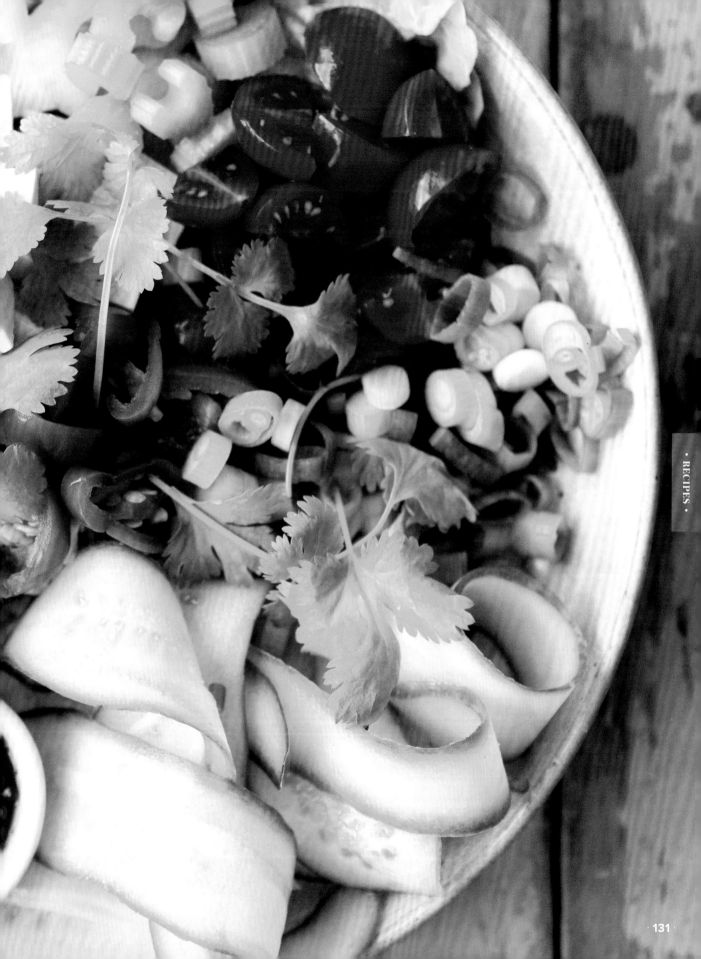

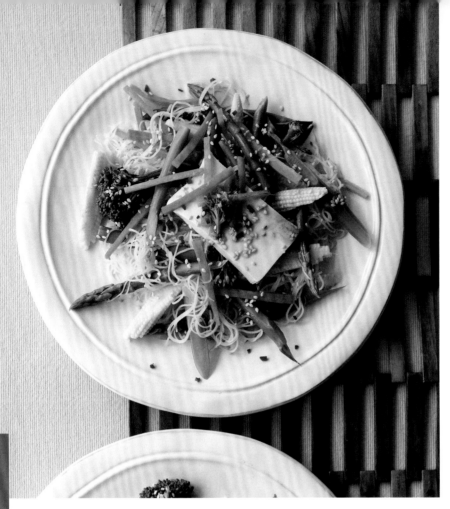

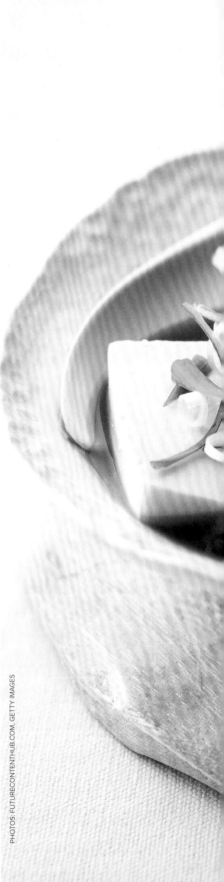

Warm Asian-style vegetable and noodle salad

Sesame oil and seeds make this salad a soothing hit.

Serves 2 • Ready in 15 mins

- **45g (1.6oz) vermicelli rice noodles**
- **1 medium carrot**
- **100g (3.5oz) baby corn**
- **200g (7oz) Tenderstem broccoli**
- **75g (2.6oz) firm tofu, sliced**
- **1tsp toasted sesame seeds**
- **½ red chilli, deseeded, finely sliced**

For the dressing:
- **Thumb-sized piece of fresh root ginger, peeled**
- **2tsp sesame oil**
- **1tbsp light soy sauce**
- **2tsp rice vinegar**

1 Put the rice noodles in a small bowl and cover with just-boiled water. Set aside for 5-10 mins, until tender, then rinse in warm water and drain well.

2 Peel the carrot and cut it into thin matchsticks. For the dressing, finely chop the ginger and combine it with the sesame oil, soy sauce and rice vinegar in a small dish.

3 Bring a pan of water to the boil and add the baby corn and broccoli. Return to the boil and cook for 1-2 mins, until just tender but still with some crunch. Drain well.

4 In a large bowl, combine the cooked noodles and vegetables with the carrot. Pour over the dressing and toss well to coat. Heap into bowls, then top with the sliced tofu and scatter over the toasted sesame seeds and sliced red chilli.

PHOTOS: FUTURECONTENTHUB.COM, GETTY IMAGES

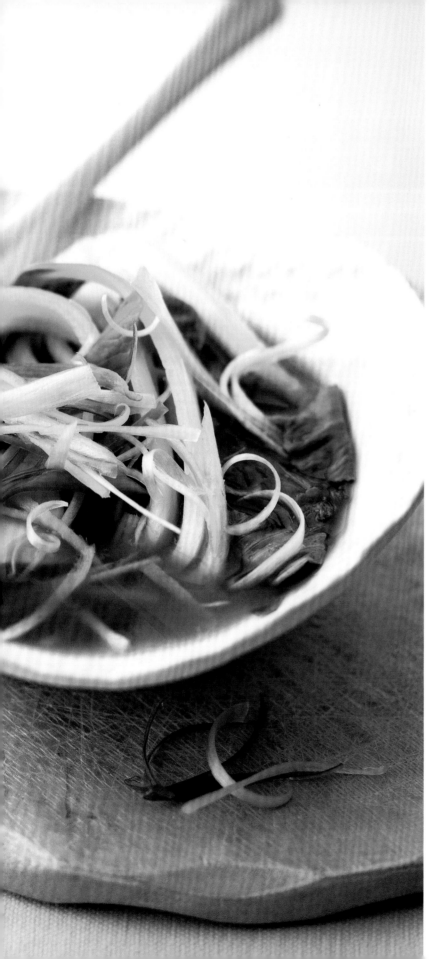

Ginger and tofu miso soup

The perfect light snack when you need a quick fix.

Serves 2 • Ready in 15 mins

- 500ml (16.9floz) vegetable stock
- 50g (1.7oz) yellow miso paste
- 10g (0.3oz) root ginger, peeled and cut into thin matchsticks
- 90g (3.1oz) baby pak choi, halved
- 150g (5.3oz) Japanese-style silken tofu, such as Yutaka, cut into cubes
- 1 spring onion, finely sliced
- 2tsp soy sauce, if liked

1 Pour the vegetable stock into a medium saucepan and bring up to a gentle simmer.
2 Put the miso paste in a small bowl, then add a spoonful of the hot stock and stir to dissolve. Stir the miso back into the pan of stock with the ginger matchsticks and simmer for 10 mins to allow the flavours to develop.
3 Add the pak choi and tofu to the soup and simmer for 1-2 mins, until the pak choi is just wilted and slightly tender, but still firm.
4 Ladle into two bowls and scatter the sliced spring onion over the top before serving. Serve with a little soy sauce for seasoning, if desired.

HEALTH TIP **Miso is a fermented food that is beneficial as it feeds your friendly gut bacteria**

Lifestyle

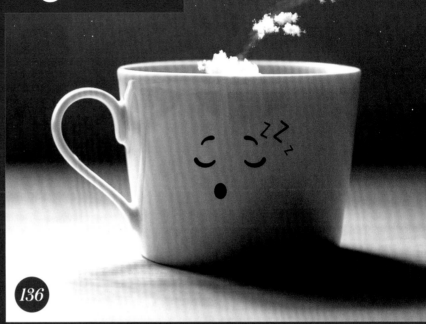

136

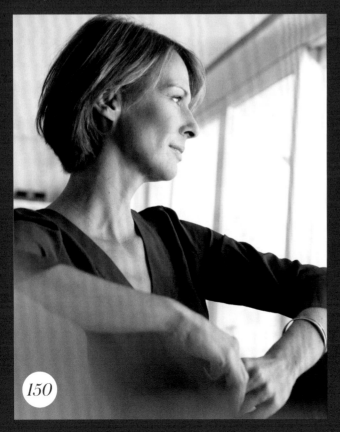

150

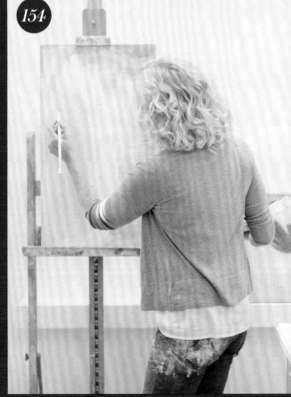

154

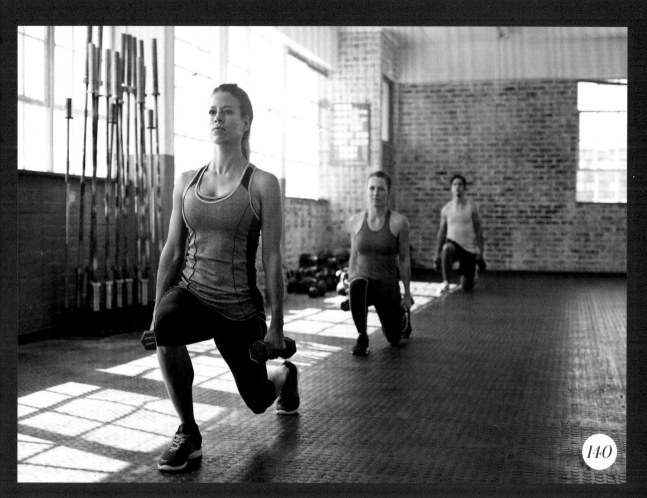

140

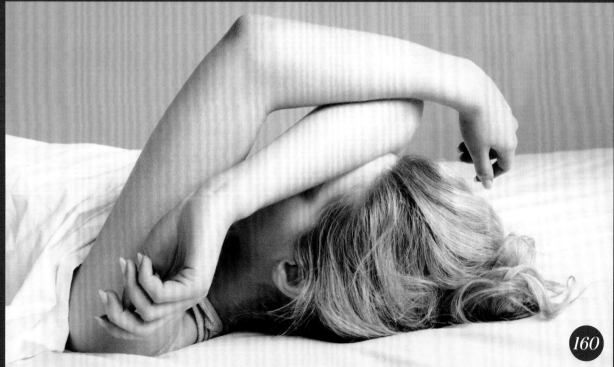

160

The A-Z of better sleep

Get a good night's rest with these
expert-backed bedtime hacks

AFTER-HOURS

When it comes to having better, healthier sleep, the first step can simply be going to bed earlier. According to a 2024 YouGov study, 27 per cent of Brits go to bed between 11.30pm and 12.30am, with 11 per cent staying up until 1am or later. However, studies show that people with an early-to-bed, early-to-rise routine are less likely to develop mental-health problems than night owls. Scientists say it takes just two weeks to tweak your body clock so that you fall asleep earlier.

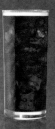

BREW UP

We already love the sleep-inducing benefits of chamomile, lavender or valerian herbal tea and of course, warm milk, but did you know that drinking tart cherry juice every day can also help you get a good night's rest. Studies show it could increase sleep time and help with insomnia.

CBD

You may have heard the hype about CBD, but how can it help you sleep? CBD oil works on the body's endocannabinoid system (ECS), which maintains stability in processes like sleep, pain perception, digestion, cognition, memory, mood and immunity. 'Clinical research has found that taking CBD oil at bedtime can alleviate insomnia and help people sleep for longer. What's more, it doesn't create the "sleep hangover" effect typical of many sleeping pills,' explains nutritionist Fiona Lawson.

DUST MITES

These pesky bedfellows – or, rather, their waste – are the most common cause of allergies in the home, giving us sleep-stealing symptoms like sneezing, stuffy nose, sore eyes and itchy skin. The average mattress contains tens of thousands of mites, and they love the warm, cosy conditions of duvets and pillows. To keep mites at bay, buy anti-allergy bedding, wash bedding at 60°C and regularly vacuum the mattress.

ENOUGH?

Everyone is different, and so is the amount of sleep we need. 'On average, a normal amount of sleep for an adult is considered to be around seven to nine hours a night,' says Dr Irshaad Ebrahim of The London Sleep Centre. This usually drops to seven to eight hours for over 65s. Use how you feel mid-morning to gauge your quota. If you're refreshed and alert, then you're probably getting enough sleep.

FITNESS FABLE

Evidence shows that adults of all ages report sleeping significantly better after doing at least 150 minutes of physical activity per week. But does the timing of your workout affect your ability to drop off? It was previously believed that strenuous exercise in the evening delayed sleep due to the rise in body temperature and the release of adrenaline, norepinephrine and cortisol, but recent findings have dismissed this idea. A study published in the *Sports Medicine* journal revealed that, as long you have an hour's recovery before bed, moderate exercise is not detrimental to a good night's sleep.

GUT HEALTH

Our gut microbiome produces and releases neurotransmitters linked to sleep, including serotonin and GABA. The sleep hormone melatonin is also produced in the gut. Some research suggests we should focus on gut health for better sleep quality. Eat prebiotic foods, such as onions, garlic, beans, pulses and lentils, or try taking a supplement.

HOT, HOT, HOT

Nearly half of menopausal women suffer with hot flushes and night sweats, according to a survey by the British Menopause Society. Taking a cool shower, keeping your bedroom cool and avoiding potential triggers such as spicy food, caffeine, nicotine and alcohol before bed can help reduce discomfort. The right bedding could also help. There are temperature-regulating bedding ranges from menopause clothing specialists that boast moisture-wicking properties and claim to keep skin drier and cooler during a night sweat.

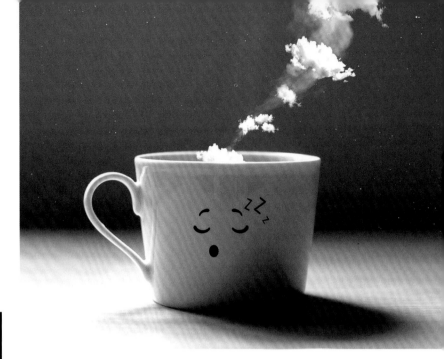

INSOMNIA

Struggle to fall asleep in under 30 minutes? Wake regularly through the night? Feel that your daytime functioning is negatively impacted? If it's been happening for over three months, this is insomnia. You don't have to accept it, though. 'CBT for insomnia is an NHS-recommended treatment which is so effective that studies show up to 85 per cent of people will see improved sleep, often in under four weeks,' says Kathryn Pinkham, founder of The Insomnia Clinic (theinsomniaclinic. co.uk). 'CBT works by tackling the physical side of the condition and re-aligning your body clock.'

JUST EAT

Sleep-friendly foods are packed with tryptophan, an amino acid that boosts sleep hormone melatonin. Turkey, milk, walnuts and pumpkin seeds are all good sources to snack on before bed.

KEEP CALM

'If you're feeling stressed before bed, focus on breathing deeply and slowly, inhaling for a count of four through the nose and exhaling for seven seconds through the mouth,' says stress and relaxation expert and motivational speaker Carole Spiers.

LIFE-SAVING

Getting adequate amounts of sleep can add years to your life and reduce the risk of obesity, heart disease, diabetes, cancer and dementia. 'Almost every known ailment...is linked in some way to poor sleep. Sleep deprivation increases our risk of developing health issues and it reduces our body's ability to cope with them,' says Professor Jason Ellis, Director of the Northumbria Centre of Sleep Research.

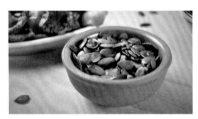

MAGIC OF MAGNESIUM

Low magnesium levels are linked to restlessness and frequent waking, and research shows a supplement can improve sleep quality. If you don't want to go the supplement route, try a handful of pumpkin seeds before bed. They are not only a good source of magnesium, but tryptophan, which also helps to promote sleep.

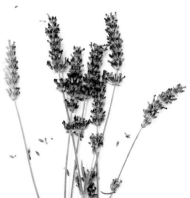

NAKED

Only one in five Brits sleeps in the buff despite there being proven advantages to the practice. Reasons to bare include better body temperature regulation, promoting a deeper sleep and faster metabolism. You'll also get a boost of oxytocin from skin-to-skin contact if sleeping with a naked partner.

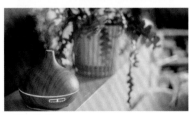

OILS

Aromatherapy oils not only make your bedroom smell good, but relieve stress and promote relaxation, allowing you to drop off faster. Try sleep-inducing classics lavender, ylang-ylang, clary sage or jasmine misted into the air via a diffuser.

POSITION POWER

Poor sleep has been linked to raised levels in brain tissue of protein deposits associated with Alzheimer's disease. Although most are swept away overnight, sleeping position can determine how effectively this happens. One study showed that brain cleansing was more effective in mice that slept on their sides than on their backs.

QUIET TIME

If you're one of the 30 per cent of people who can't snooze in silence, download the **noisli app (noisli.com app)**. The soothing audio includes white, pink and brown noise – everything from a whirring fan to forest noise with birdsong – to help you unwind and nod off gradually.

TENSION

If you lie in bed with a tensed-up body and jaw, your sleep will suffer. 'To relax, squeeze the muscles in your feet, hold, then release; move up through your body doing the same until you reach the top of the head,' suggests Claire Dale and Patricia Peyton, authors of *Physical Intelligence*.

RECOVERING SLEEP

Don't fret about occasional sleep deprivation, as it's lighter sleep that's lost. 'Nearly half of sleep consists of lightsleep, a quarter of deep sleep and a quarter of rapid eye movement (REM) sleep. If you lose sleep one night, deep and REM sleep increases the next,' says Dr Chris Idzikowski, author of *Sleep Well*.

URINARY URGE

One in 10 people under 45 has to urinate in the night, and this increases with age. Needing a wee more than twice at night is called nocturia and can be caused by diabetes, sleep apnoea, hormonal changes, a weak pelvic floor or too much fluid before bed. If nocturia persists, see your GP to rule out a UTI.

SNORING

There are approximately 15 million snorers in the UK, according to the British Snoring & Sleep Apnoea Association. Anti-snore pillows claim to reduce the rumbles thanks to their shape. These pillows are designed to optimise head and neck position to improve breathing by keeping your airways open as you sleep.

VIVID DREAMS

Ever wondered why we have crazy and memorable dreams? Around 25 per cent of our night's sleep is spent in rapid eye movement (REM), the sleep stage important for learning and memory. Because brain activity is similar to that of being awake during REM, it's when we dream intensely, according to scientists. Stress, sleep deprivation, medication and hormone fluctuations have all been linked to more vivid dreams says the Sleep Council.

WIND-DOWN & WAKE-UP

Use light therapy to help you fall asleep faster and wake up feeling more refreshed. Sleep and wake-up lamps are designed to help you wind down before bed and wake up ready for the day ahead. You can use different settings to simulate the rising and setting of the sun. By gradually dimming the light in the evening and gradually brightening the light in the morning your body will go to sleep and wake up more naturally so that you feel more rested.

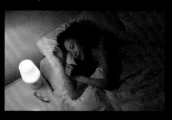

XEROSTOMIA

This is the medical term for a dry mouth. Saliva production can decrease by 40 per cent as we age, and fluctuating hormones during menopause may exacerbate things. A dry mouth can disturb sleep and affect tooth and gum health. Drinking plenty during the day, sleeping with a humidifier and avoiding alcohol-based mouthwash will all help.

YESTERNIGHT

'If you're lying awake feeling the hours slip away, turn the clock away or move it to a different room if you can. Seeing time move on will increase your anxiety and keep you awake longer,' says Carole Spiers.

ZINC

This essential mineral and antioxidant is key for sleep regulation. For a restorative night's sleep, try taking a zinc supplement or make sure your diet is rich in zinc with plenty of shellfish, beef and pork or nuts and seeds.

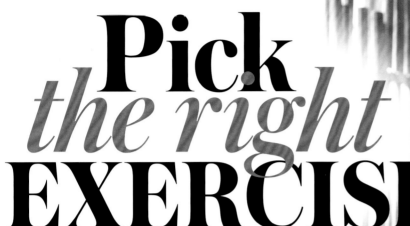

Pick *the right* EXERCISE

It's important that you enjoy your fitness activities, so choose something you like to do

There is no one form of exercise that is better than another. There are lots of different types of exercise that you can choose from. If you prefer something low-impact and gentle but that gets your heart rate up a little, consider walking or swimming. If you're looking for something to work both the mind and body, then things like yoga, Pilates and martial arts are great options. If you want to get outside in the fresh air, then look at cycling, running or outdoor bootcamps. And if you like the idea of being among other like-minded people and trying something new, there is a plethora of gym classes to get involved with.

Exercise is simply moving your body in some way, getting your heart rate up and warming your body. There really is something for everyone. You might think you 'hate' exercise, but this could be because you haven't found the right thing for you yet. It's so important that you enjoy the type of exercise you do; it will encourage and motivate you to do it more often and get better results.

If you don't want to join a gym or go for a run, then think outside the box. Consider activities like paddleboarding or kayaking, which are great forms of exercise as they use your core, challenge your balance and raise your heart rate.

Any form of exercise counts, so even if you walk faster on the school run, take the stairs more often, get off the bus a few stops early or jump about on a trampoline, it's all part of your fitness journey.

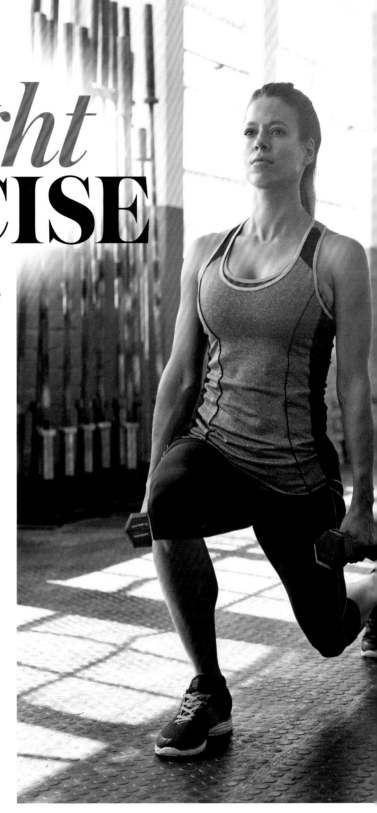

What's right for you?

IF YOU'RE COMPETITIVE
✣ If you enjoy pushing yourself and like winning, why not consider trying a team sport? Things like football, netball, hockey, rugby and tennis doubles are available in most areas for all levels. There is always the chance to improve your game, play matches and make the most of that competitive streak.

IF YOU LIKE VARIETY
✣ Consider a bootcamp or circuits class, which challenges you to move from station to station performing lots of different exercises. There is no chance to get bored as you are continually switching it up.

IF YOU'RE SHORT OF TIME
✣ When time is tight, interval training is your perfect go-to activity. High-Intensity Interval Training (HIIT) is a type of exercise that involves hard work for a short period of time, with a rest in between sets. You can complete a workout in just 20 minutes and feel great!

IF YOU HAVE LIMITED FUNDS
✣ Running is a great way to get fit quickly without spending too much. As long as you have some decent trainers, you can start running. If your office has a shower, you could even combine running with your commute to save money on travel too.

IF YOU LOVE THE OUTDOORS
✣ Get those walking boots on and start hiking! Exploring rural trails can be a great way to see the country, as well as get fit. As long as you have the right kit, you can do it all year round and increase the length and elevation of your hikes to push your fitness.

IF YOU LIKE MAKING NEW FRIENDS
✣ Dancing is a great way to make friends in your local area. Whether you fancy ballroom or salsa, Zumba or line dancing, there are plenty of styles for you to try to meet like-minded people along the way.

IF YOU STRUGGLE TO GET MOTIVATED
✣ Motivation can be hard to come by, especially when there are so many distractions in life. Try pre-booking classes or gym sessions in advance, so that you have them in your diary. There's something about having paid for a class that helps motivate you to stick with it.

IF YOU LACK CONFIDENCE
✣ Start in the comfort of your own home by investing in a few workout DVDs or finding some workouts on the internet. This will help you build the confidence to perform exercises correctly, which might lead to you joining public classes in time.

TRY BEFORE YOU BUY
Many clubs, groups, gyms or pools will have the option of a free trial so you can give something a go before committing to it. This can be a good way of exploring your options and seeing what you like.

Running & walking

POP UP AT PARKRUN
If you can run, walk or even combine both over 5K, why not try your local parkrun? There are hundreds of these events across the country, taking place every Saturday morning. They are free to attend and open to all.

Running and walking are the most natural forms of exercise that you can do. We all walk every single day, even if it's just from A to B. You don't need any fancy equipment to start walking, you don't need a gym membership and you can adapt it to suit any amount of time that you have.

Walking is very underrated as a form of exercise, but it is the perfect place to start. The idea is to walk slightly faster than your normal walking pace so that you raise your heart rate a little. Try to fit extra steps into your day on a regular basis, such as walking to work if you can, or planning a walk after dinner to shake off the day. Start with just 15 minutes and build up from there. You can challenge yourself by walking in different environments, such as off-road or uphill, and it's easy to get family members and friends involved. Many areas will offer health walks that are specifically designed to help you get fit through walking.

If you want to move a bit faster, you might want to take up running. If you have never run before, then consider a Couch to 5K style programme, of which there are a few to pick from. These start with a walk-and-run approach, with set intervals that build up week on week until you can, over time, run a 5K distance. If you run a little already, you might want to follow a plan designed to help you hit your next milestone distance or improve your pace.

You can run or walk on a treadmill in the gym or at home if you prefer, but getting outside will give you more health and fitness benefits. You'll be out in the fresh air, and your body works harder to adapt to the changing terrain, camber and bends.

Track your steps

If you're interested in using walking as your choice of exercise, invest in a method of tracking steps, such as a pedometer, phone app or activity watch. You can set yourself goals on how many steps you want to walk in a day, and you can slowly increase this goal as you get fitter. It can be a great way of keeping your motivation up.

'If you run, you are a runner. It doesn't matter how fast or how far'
– John Bingham, marathon runner

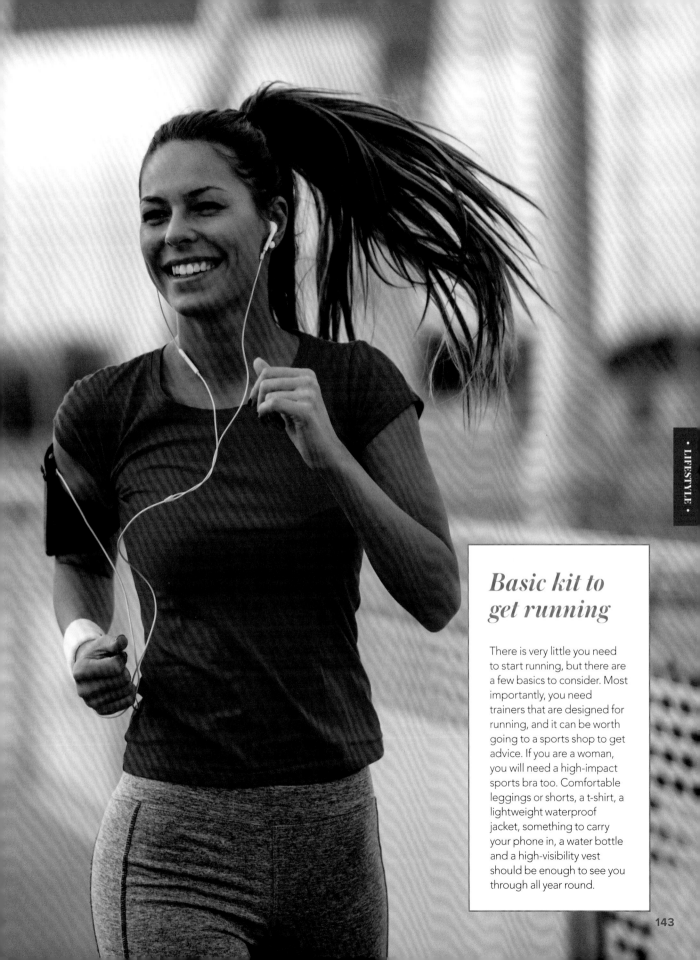

Basic kit to get running

There is very little you need to start running, but there are a few basics to consider. Most importantly, you need trainers that are designed for running, and it can be worth going to a sports shop to get advice. If you are a woman, you will need a high-impact sports bra too. Comfortable leggings or shorts, a t-shirt, a lightweight waterproof jacket, something to carry your phone in, a water bottle and a high-visibility vest should be enough to see you through all year round.

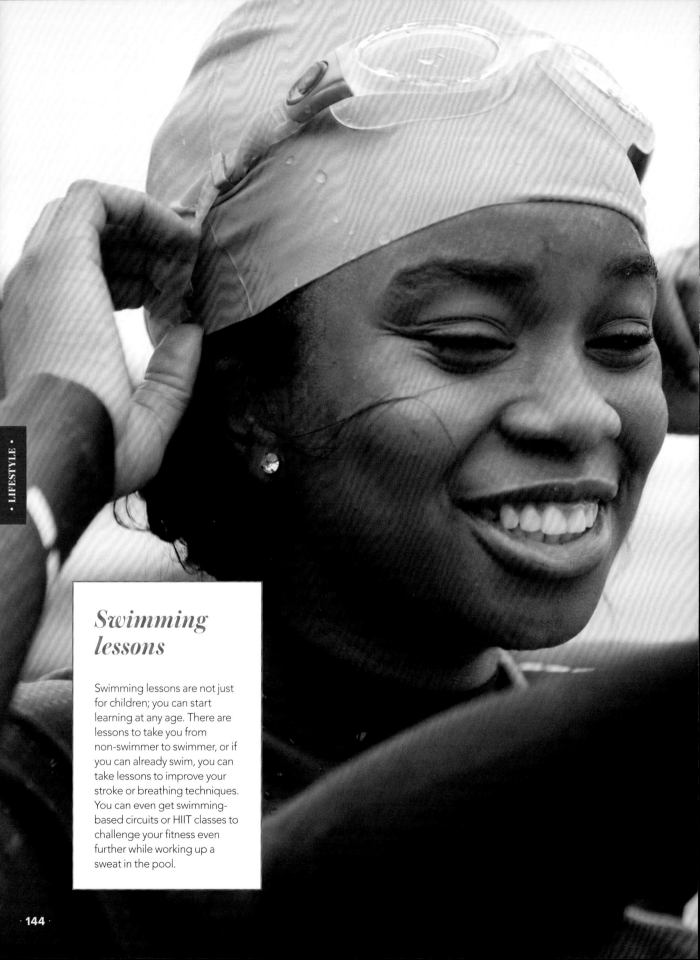

Swimming lessons

Swimming lessons are not just for children; you can start learning at any age. There are lessons to take you from non-swimmer to swimmer, or if you can already swim, you can take lessons to improve your stroke or breathing techniques. You can even get swimming-based circuits or HIIT classes to challenge your fitness even further while working up a sweat in the pool.

Ever considered a triathlon? It's not just for the super fit or elite! Beginner triathlon events often include a pool swim rather than in the sea. You can start with a Super Sprint, which is a 300-metre swim, 8K bike ride and 2K run, then build up to longer distances.

Swimming & cycling

Here are two amazing low-impact exercises you can do. You might already use a bike on a casual basis, or it may have been years since you last got on one, but cycling is a great form of exercise. It's endlessly adaptable to suit your ability and preferences.

You can use a bike to commute to work – great for your wallet, your fitness and the planet! There are lots of cycling groups around too, which cater for those who want more structure with a training plan, or those who want group rides with like-minded people on a more leisurely basis. You may prefer to cycle off-road or on a traffic-free cycle path. There are plenty of good cycling networks that offer both long- and short-distance routes, so take a look to see what paths there are near you.

You could also improve your cycling fitness by going to spinning classes at the gym. These are held on static bikes with different resistance levels to simulate hills. They are high-intensity classes, so you'll burn lots of calories!

If you prefer to be in the water rather than on the roads, then consider swimming. This can be a great option if you want to focus on cardiovascular fitness. Swimming is a low-impact activity, so it's easy on the joints and good for those who may struggle with injury. You can increase your stroke speed to raise your heart rate, or go for the endurance option and see how many lengths you can manage at a slower pace. Check out

Cycle safe

If you've not been on the roads for a while, you should consider a cycle safety course before getting on your bike. These courses offer a refresher on things like how to switch lanes, signal, turn across traffic, use roundabouts and keep a safe distance between yourself and vehicles. This can help to build your confidence on the roads and help you to stay safe.

your local pool timetable – you can usually find adults-only sessions, which can be good if you don't want kids jumping in around you. Or, if you have children, you can all go together and make it a fun way to work out as a family.

You're not limited to the pool either. Wild and outdoor swimming is gaining popularity. If it's your first time, stick to designated lakes or lidos to get used to it. Join an outdoor swimming group to pick up hints and tips, and discover safe places to swim. If you're swimming in the sea, don't forget the golden rule – swim where the lifeguards are!

• LIFESTYLE •

145

The gym & group training

Got a gym membership that you never use? Well, now is the time to change that. The gym offers so many different possibilities and there is sure to be something that suits you.

For a start, there is the gym itself. It can be quite an intimidating environment at first, with every exercise machine under the sun available to use, so don't be afraid to ask for an induction or a re-induction so that a member of staff can show you how to use all the equipment properly. It can help to have a proper workout plan to follow, so you don't just flit from machine to machine. The gym staff should be able to help with this, but you could always hire a personal trainer for a few sessions to help you get confident with it.

Think about what you want to get out of your gym sessions. It might be that you want to work solely on strength to complement the fat-burning cardio work that you already do, or perhaps you would prefer a well-balanced programme that incorporates both cardio and strength work.

Don't be afraid of the free weights area either. You don't have to be building big muscles to go here. There are plenty of bodyweight and free weight exercises that you can try, which will help you to build lean muscle, improve your fitness and burn calories. If you're unsure, see if your gym offers any gym floor classes. These are small classes, of usually no more than six people, that use the equipment in the gym itself to give you a good workout. As they are run by an instructor, you can be sure that you are doing it properly.

It's also worth taking a look at the class timetable in your gym. There are so many forms of group training – including things like aerobics, boxing-based classes, interval workouts, circuits, stretch classes – that there is bound to be something for you.

Outdoor and home gyms

There are alternatives to using your local gym. If you have the space, you could set up a small gym at home so you can work out at any time. You don't need much – a mat, a few different weights and some resistance bands is a good start, and you can add more kit as you go. In many parks you will also find small, free-to-use outdoor gyms. These are often based on traditional gym machines powered with your bodyweight, and are a brilliant way to get fit.

'Don't be afraid to ask for an induction or a re-induction so that a member of staff can show you how to use all the equipment properly'

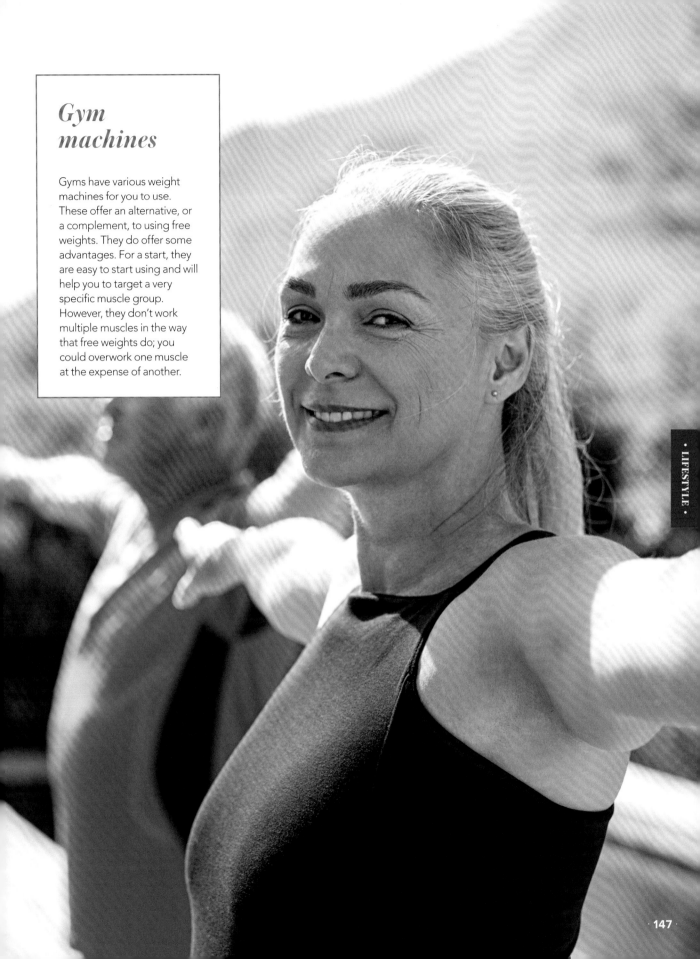

Gym machines

Gyms have various weight machines for you to use. These offer an alternative, or a complement, to using free weights. They do offer some advantages. For a start, they are easy to start using and will help you to target a very specific muscle group. However, they don't work multiple muscles in the way that free weights do; you could overwork one muscle at the expense of another.

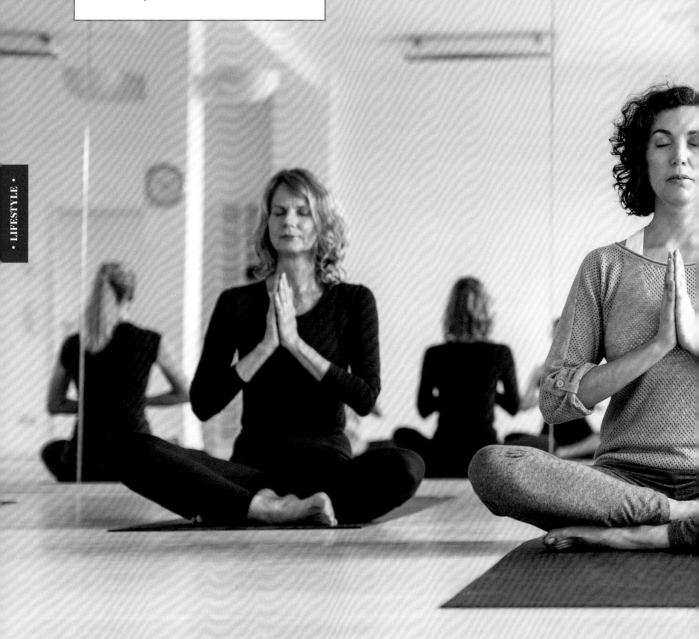

And relax...

The relaxation element at the end of a yoga or Pilates class can take some getting used to, especially if you're not one for lying still or meditating, but it's a great skill to learn and has a whole host of benefits. Spending a few minutes relaxing after a workout, listening to the silence or working through a guided meditation helps your mental wellbeing. The more you do it, the easier it will become.

Yoga & Pilates

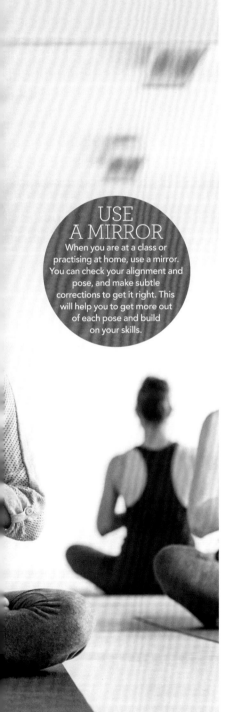

Yoga and Pilates are often put together, and while they are similar in many ways, they are also quite different.

Yoga is an ancient form of exercise, which challenges you to move from pose to pose while controlling your breathing. The poses are designed to help build your strength, flexibility and fitness, while the breathing techniques can help you to practise mindfulness and improve mental wellbeing.

There are lots of different types of yoga that you can try. They range in difficulty from gentle beginners' classes, where you will spend more time in each pose in order to learn proper technique, to more dynamic classes that get your heart rate up by moving from one pose to another more quickly. There are lots of variations and progressions for each pose, which means that you can continue to challenge yourself over and over again.

Pilates, however, is relatively modern. It was invented by Joseph Pilates, who brought it into the USA when he moved there from Germany in the 1920s. Pilates works to improve core strength and help you to become more aware of how the body connects. It can be adapted for

> '*Yoga means addition — addition of energy, strength and beauty to body, mind and soul*'
> — *Amit Ray, author*

Home vs classes

You can get plenty of apps, DVDs and online videos to guide you through yoga or Pilates routines. This can be useful to keep your workouts going at home, it's easy to fit into your day and very useful if you're away from home. However, it is also useful to initially attend some classes if you can, as the instructor can help you to get your posture and poses right, so that you get the most out of your workouts.

people of all ages and abilities, and can be quite challenging, even if you are fit. It helps you to develop strength, which can also help to protect from injury. It is also possible to use different equipment, like resistance bands, to adapt exercises.

Because both Pilates and yoga provide similar low-impact, strength-building benefits, there are now classes that bring the two together into combined workouts. PIYO, for example, is a fast-moving, high-intensity workout that uses both yoga and Pilates principles in a cardio workout. Body Balance combines Pilates, yoga and Tai Chi, and focuses on working the whole body one area at a time, ending with a chance to relax and meditate. See what's on offer at your local gym.

Soothe
your
stress

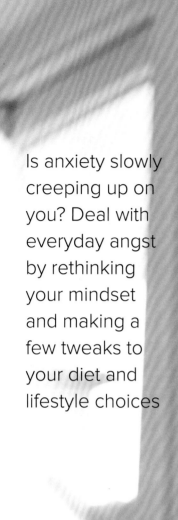

Is anxiety slowly creeping up on you? Deal with everyday angst by rethinking your mindset and making a few tweaks to your diet and lifestyle choices

The unprecedented unfolding of the years following the 2020 pandemic resulted in a roller coaster of negative emotions for many of us. If you felt low as a result, you're not alone – nearly half of all British adults experienced high levels of anxiety during lockdown. GP Dr Folusha Oluwajana says: 'It's normal to be stressed and scared during a crisis but the way we deal with these feelings can have huge effects on our mental health.

'When our brains decide that a stressful event is occurring, the sympathetic nervous system is stimulated; known as fight or flight response, to keep the body at a steady state of equilibrium. In response to a stress, the brain stimulates this part of the nervous system, which then activates the adrenal glands.'

On a physical level, fight or flight results in faster breathing and increased blood pressure. Your sense of pain is reduced, and strength increased.

'In addition, the brain releases hormones that stimulate the adrenal glands to release the stress hormone cortisol, which enhances the effects of adrenaline by releasing more glucose,' says Dr Oluwajana. 'It also shuts down systems that are nonessential to the stress response, such as the digestive and reproductive systems.'

In the short-term, this stress response isn't a worry; chronic stress, however, can be detrimental.

'Persistently high glucose levels can lead to insulin resistance and type 2 diabetes. Excess cortisol can lead to digestive issues and flare-ups of conditions such as irritable bowel syndrome,' says Dr Oluwajana.

Plus, you may be more prone to infections and injury; persistently raised cortisol levels suppress the immune system and promote muscle and protein breakdown. The production of 'happy hormone' serotonin can also be altered leading to irritability, disturbed sleep and mental health disorders. Here we share some of the biggest stress culprits and suggest ways to feel more serene and less stressed.

STRESS CULPRIT: NIGHT TIME PANIC

The evening is often the time when anxiety rears its ugly head. If you've been frantically juggling tasks throughout the day and haven't really had a moment to pause, it's these night time hours when anxiety can strike. You might find it difficult to get to sleep, or lie awake at 3am stressing about everything from work deadlines to your relationship. According to The Sleep Charity 37 per cent of us suffer from sleepless nights or insomnia. 'Fragmented sleep is associated with persistently raised cortisol levels throughout the day. This can cause a vicious cycle of stress, raised cortisol levels and sleep disturbance,' believes Dr Oluwajana.

STRESS-SOOTHING PLAN:

Practical steps such as avoiding digital devices and sticking to a regular nightly routine where you go to bed at the same time can help to improve sleep quality, and thankfully your diet can also play a part. A study published in the *Journal of Clinical Sleep Medicine* found that diets that are low in fibre and high in saturated fat and sugar are linked to poorer sleep with less time in the restore phase of sleep, known as slow-wave sleep. Frequent night-time awakenings can also alter appetite hormones such as leptin and ghrelin, which can cause cravings and increased appetite. To counteract these effects, eat more sleep-friendly foods. These include magnesium-packed leafy greens and tryptophan-rich chickpeas, turkey and milk.

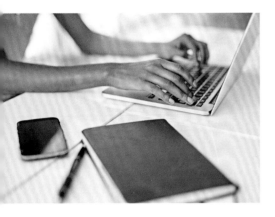

STRESS CULPRIT: WORKING FROM HOME

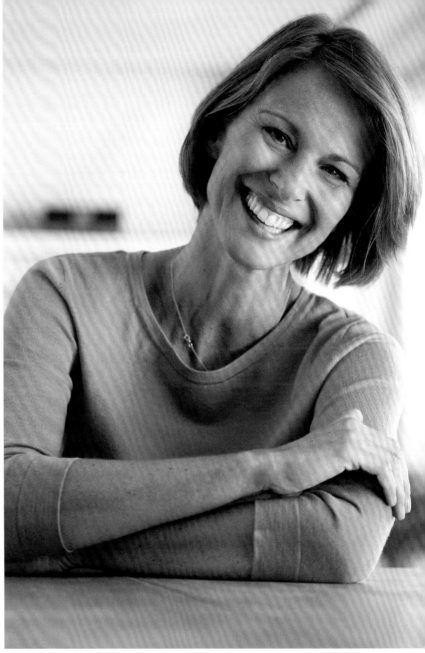

The ripple effects of the unprecedented pandemic left many of us feeling a lack of control. The sense of uncertainty in the air, financial constraints, health concerns and in some cases the after effects of bereavement contributed to rising levels of stress; in fact a whopping 25 million of us admitted drowning in anxiety throughout lockdown according to a report by the Office of National Statistics.

Many of us had to re-think the way we work, which brought its own unique challenges. While there were no intimidating board meetings or lengthy commute to contend with, for many of us working from home meant juggling our day-to-day work schedules with home life, while coping with the pressure of remaining productive.

Following the pandemic, many companies reassessed the need for offices, which meant more and more people started to work from home either full or part-time. Being holed up at home can certainly take its toll on our health, especially when the lines between work and personal life are so blurred.

STRESS-SOOTHING PLAN:

Striving for a good work-life balance is super-important when working from home to avoid being too stressed. This means sticking to a clear schedule, which marks the beginning of the working day, as well as the end – avoiding replying to emails or finishing a work project when you should officially be 'out of the office'.

Designate a space in your home as your work zone; this should be separate from where you eat and where you sleep and should be organised and calm.

Your diet also plays a crucial role when you're working from home. It can be tempting to reach for snacks around the clock, but this will just leave you feeling lethargic and sluggish. Having a strict working day where you start work at say 9am and finish at 5pm will allow you to slot in three regular meals, one mid-morning and one mid-afternoon snack. Breakfast is the most crucial consideration here, as smart eating in the morning will set up your energy levels and your mood for the entire day. A protein and complex carbohydrate-based breakfast such as oats with seeds and berries or poached eggs on wholemeal toast helps to keep blood sugar levels even so that you don't run on empty. Don't forget to drink water and take short breaks throughout the day too.

WORDS: LOUISE PYNE. PHOTOS (POSED BY MODELS): GETTY

STRESS CULPRIT: OVER TRAINING

Physical activity is vital for mental health and the rush of endorphins when we get moving massively improves our feel-good factor, something that most of us need now more than ever. On the flip side however, too much exercise can have adverse health effects. Prolonged high intensity exercise without adequate rest time in between sessions can throw your body out of kilter resulting in excess cortisol and higher levels of inflammation, impacting everything from immunity to energy. 'This is known as over training syndrome, and signs to look out for include decreased performance, increased perceived effort, prolonged muscle soreness and fatigue after exercise, recurrent injury or illness, sleep disturbance, irritability and low mood,' says Dr Oluwajana.

STRESS-SOOTHING PLAN:

Listening to your body's needs is the best way to manage exercise-induced stress. 'The over-training threshold is different for everyone so you need to pay attention to how your body is coping, while ensuring that you are getting adequate sleep, water and nutrients,' she adds.

You might need to mix up your workouts, weaving in high-intensity runs with rolling out your yoga mat or going for long walks to mindfully engage in the present moment and reduce stress. Include more immunity-boosting foods in your diet. These include vitamin C-rich orange and grapefruit, which contain special flavonoid compounds to help increase immune system activity, and zinc-packed pumpkin seeds and shellfish to help reduce any inflammation in your cells.

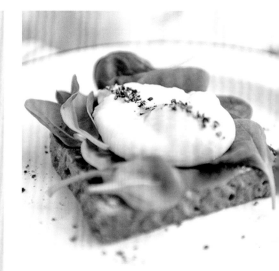

STRESS CULPRIT: MICROMANAGING YOUR DIET

You might count calories or skip meals in a bid to see the number on the scales drop, but constant dieting can lead to emotional and physical stress. The chronic stress of yo-yo dieting can ignite flight or fight mode, leading to anxiety and irritability. 'You'll be lacking in vital nutrients and a nutrient-deficient diet can pose a form of stress on the body. Chronic stress can impair the absorption and deplete stores of essential vitamins, potentially leading to deficiencies,' explains Dr Oluwajana.

STRESS-SOOTHING PLAN:

If you're not eating enough in the day, you'll have reduced levels of important nutrients and lower levels of neurotransmitters. To ensure you're getting enough nutrients, fill half your plate with a variety of veg (peppers, spinach, broccoli), a quarter of your plate with lean protein (chicken, tofu or legumes), and the rest with complex carbohydrates (such as wholegrain rice or sweet potato), and healthy fats such as olive oil, avocado, nuts and seeds. This ensures you're getting a range of healthy nutrients to sustain energy and mood without having to rely on restrictive calorie counting.

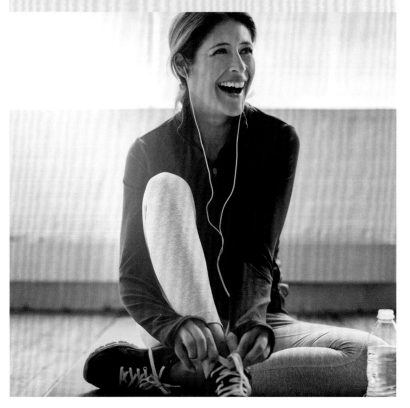

Learning to
RELA

Discovering a new way of self-soothing – be it with an activity or natural medication – can swiftly reduce stress levels. So what will suit you best?

Relaxation is an essential addition to our wellbeing toolkit, but it's not always easy to accomplish, especially in challenging circumstances. But learning to do it right could give your health a much-needed boost.

'Relaxation is vital to our health and wellbeing, as well as our immune function,' says natural health and wellness expert Dr Tim Bond. 'Researchers at Harvard Medical School discovered that in people practising relaxation methods, such as yoga and meditation, far more "disease-fighting genes" were active, compared to those who didn't practise. In particular, they found genes were switched on that help to protect from disorders such as pain, infertility, high blood pressure and even rheumatoid arthritis.'

And that's not all. The art of relaxation also drives higher levels of feel-good chemicals, such as serotonin and growth hormones, which repair cells and tissue. 'In essence, relaxation has virtually the opposite effect to stress, lowering heart rate, boosting immunity and enabling the body to thrive,' says Dr Bond. 'An example is when women menstruate, they often find taking a long bath or doing some gentle relaxation exercises helps their general wellbeing.'

Sounds great, but our hectic lives often prevent us from finding – and utilising – what's best for us. In order to move away from the sympathetic (fight or flight) response and activate the parasympathetic (rest and digest) response, we must trust our instincts and choose what produces the most satisfaction. 'It's about finding out what's right for you,' says Dr Megan Jones Bell, chief science officer at Headspace (headspace.com). 'Breathing can be a powerful way to help us reset and activate our natural relaxation response, so one of the easiest and most accessible ways for anyone to relax, in any setting, environment or activity, is to focus on the breath.'

As well as spending time in nature, playing with animals, getting a massage, and praying or meditating, here are some quick and effective ways to put you back on the path to wellness.

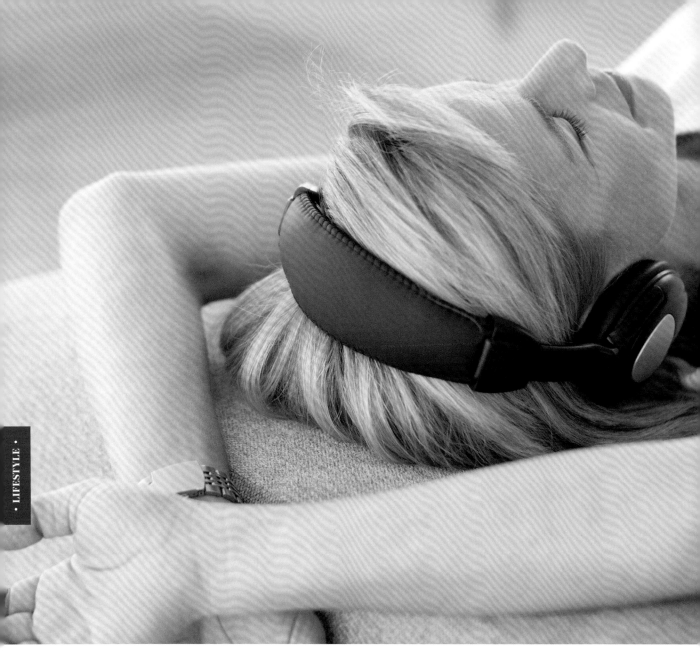

The art of...
creating

Creating can be anything, from colouring in, to crafts or jigsaw puzzles. These forms of active meditation allow us to settle our overworked brains. 'Art has the power to heal, increase wellbeing and reduce anxiety. Researchers liken [it] to exercise for the brain, and studies consistently show that creating art helps individuals cope with stressful and difficult situations,' says Scott Phillips, co-founder of Rise Art (riseart.com).

Even doodling is beneficial. Writing in *Psychology Today* (psychologytoday.com), Cathy Malchiodi, PhD, says: 'The wonderful thing about doodling is that it is a whole-brain activity – self-soothing, satisfying, exploratory and mindful.'

The art of...
yogic breathing

Brighton-based yoga practitioner Danny Griffiths (yoga-fit.co.uk) recommends alternate nostril breathing, called nadi shodhana pranayama. It activates the parasympathetic response, strengthening the immune system and providing quick relief from stress.

She says, 'I do this before classes, as I find it really relaxing and calming. It's meant to balance the "ida" and "pingala" nadis (channels) or the yin and the yang.' Explaining how to do it, she says, 'Sit up straight in a cross-legged position with your left hand resting on your thigh, exhale completely then use your right thumb to close your right nostril. Inhale for 4 to 5 seconds through your left

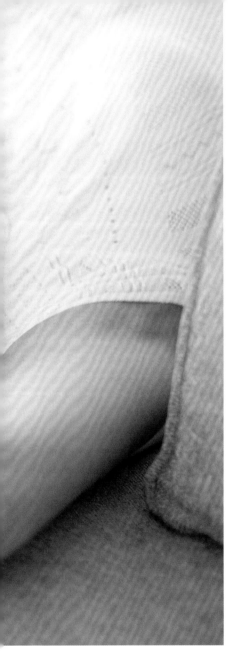

The art of... *sound therapy*

Sound therapy, such as drumming, singing, chanting and gong baths, has been used for centuries to help people enter a more relaxed, meditative state and promote wellbeing and healing. Now, thanks to modern technology, there's a new-ish kid on the block – binaural beats.

Through headphones, listeners receive a different sound frequency to each ear, which the brain interprets as a particular rhythmic frequency. These sounds create specific neural responses that, depending on the frequency, induce one of five brainwave states that can aid sleep and ease pain (delta brainwaves), help you relax or meditate (theta), reduce stress (alpha), improve concentration and focus (beta), and enhance memory (gamma).

Look up binaural beats on YouTube or sign in to Spotify (spotify.com/uk) and search for 'the most relaxing songs ever according to science'. Backed by neuroscientists, it's so effective that it's strongly recommended you don't drive while tuning in.

---

nostril then close this nostril with your ring finger and exhale for 4 to 5 seconds through your right nostril. Inhale through the right nostril then close it with your thumb and breathe out through the left nostril. Repeat for 3 to 5 minutes. Finish on the left nostril.'

While this type of breathing can be done at any time, it's worth combining with yoga. 'Yoga is more of a work-in than work-out,' says Danny. 'Classes are meditative as we move from posture to posture, and for some students it's the only time they can switch off. After concentrating on how the body feels in

the moment, there's no denying the state of relaxation at the end of practice.'

The art of... *organising*

If your mum ever said 'tidy house, tidy mind', she probably wasn't just trying to persuade you to clean your room – the chances are she recognised the positive effects of an ordered environment. And, with the rise in popularity of the staycation in the UK, it's more important than ever to create a Zen home.

Research has shown that working up a sweat while cleaning your house can actually help to improve your mental health and boost your mood, while Japanese author and organising consultant Marie Kondo waxes lyrical about how a home should be 'a comfortable environment, a space that feels good to be in, a place where you can relax' in her bestselling book *The Life-Changing Magic of Tidying Up*.

'With the rise in popularity of the staycation, it's important to create a Zen home'

The art of... *ASMR*

For those who enjoy Autonomous Sensory Meridian Response (ASMR), the experience can be nothing short of profound. ASMR enthusiasts love the de-stressing effects of listening to sounds, such as whispering, eating, a cat purring or rainfall, or by watching kinetic sand or soap being sliced, or even pimples being popped.

The theory behind these stimuli is the release of feel-good chemicals – endorphins, dopamine, oxytocin and

DO YOU SUFFER FROM RELAXATION REMORSE?

Dr Christine Langhoff, Clinical Psychologist and Director of Circle Psychology Partners in south London (circlepsychology partners.co.uk), explains why we sometimes feel guilty just taking it easy...

'It can come from many places, including our upbringing, schooling, religion, the media and cultural expectations,' says Dr Langhoff.

'Our lives have become increasingly busy with both real and perceived pressures that, for many, have led to perfectionism.

'Whilst striving for high standards is not a bad thing, overly focusing on them increases stress levels and the pressure on ourselves.'

Christine's tips:

✦ Remember that relaxing is an important part of staying physically and mentally healthy.
✦ What we find relaxing is subjective – what works for you may not for another. Bear this in mind if you tend to compare yourself to others.
✦ Be kind to yourself. It can be hard – but, with practice, relaxing becomes easier.
✦ Set aside allocated time to relax, even if you feel that you 'don't deserve it' or 'have too much to do'. This could be anything from taking a yoga class to ensuring that you take regular short breaks.

'ASMR enthusiasts love the de-stressing effects of sounds, such as whispering'

serotonin – into our bodies, which decrease stress and aid relaxation and sleep. 'ASMR is consistently helpful at bringing comfort, peace and calmness to busy brains when an overactive mind is preventing a desired feeling of calmness. While it can't cure or prevent any form of illness, it may help reduce feelings of stress or sleeplessness,' explains Dr Craig Richard, founder of ASMR University (asmruniversity.com).

The art of... *natural self-medicating with cannabidiol*

If you self-medicate with alcohol or drugs, try a natural approach instead – it's better for your body and mental state. 'Quality, tested CBD [cannabidiol] oil like DragonflyCBD (dragonflycbd. com) has been found to bust anxiety and stress and help a user, together with other self-care tips, to get to that deep relaxation state,' explains Dr Bond. 'Evidence from studies have shown that CBD has anti-anxiety effects, may regulate learned fear, and appears to reduce the cardiovascular response to models of stress and reduce resting blood pressure,' he adds.

The art of... *salt bathing*

Salt baths have long been regarded as an elixir to combat stress and encourage relaxation, and the secret lies in magnesium. 'Individuals who

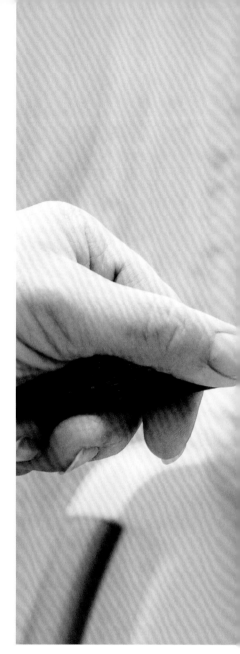

suffer with mental-health illnesses have been found to have lower platelet serotonin levels,' explains Karen Davis, Westlab Chief Pharmacist (westlabsalts. co.uk). 'There are different ways to increase serotonin, including magnesium intake,' she adds. 'This is best absorbed through the skin.'

That's why a long soak in a bath filled with salts rich in magnesium, such as Dead Sea, Epsom or Himalayan salts, is advised. 'This will not only help to calm and de-stress the mind and body, but also improve mood,' Karen explains.

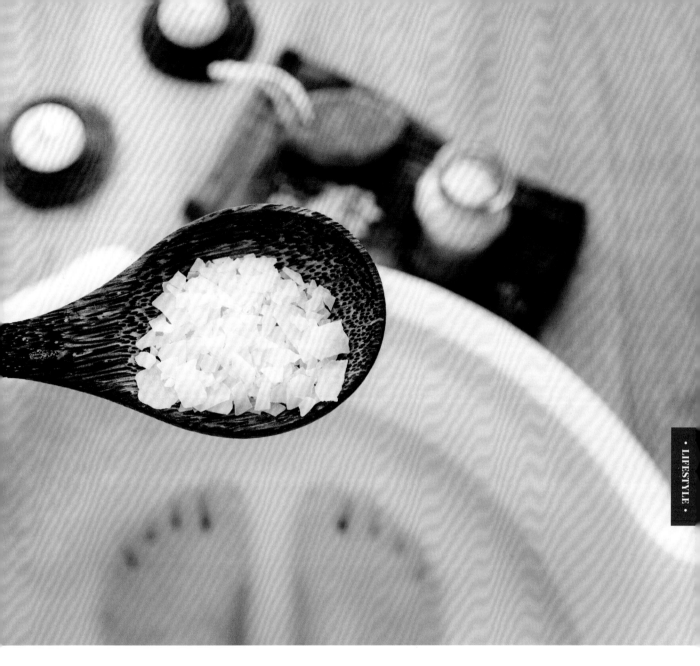

The art of...
everyday mindfulness

Contrary to popular belief, mindfulness isn't about sitting quietly and meditating. 'We can introduce relaxation into our daily life by simply trying to be more mindful in our everyday tasks,' explains Dr Jones Bell. 'This could be as simple as mindful hand-washing, making a cup of tea or taking moments to pause and check in with yourself. Rather than getting lost in the frustration of a task, acknowledge it, accept it, sit with it, focus on your breathing and bring your attention back to how you're feeling and why. This will help you be intentional in every interaction and can bring about a more relaxed state of being,' she says.

The art of...
neo-Luddism

For those of us attached to our phones and laptops, a little neo-Luddism goes a long way, because if you're constantly distracted by your phone or email you'll never be able to relax. Neo-Luddites reject modern technology and so can you. 'Give it a go, even for an hour, and see what difference it makes,' says burnout coach Rosie Millen (missnutritionist.com). 'We live in a comparative age, which is not healthy. From the moment we wake up to the moment we go to bed we are reminded of what everyone is doing and achieving in every 24-hour window. This further emphasises the need to switch off to get in touch with real life.'

WORDS: DEBRA WATERS. PHOTOS (POSED BY MODELS): GETTY

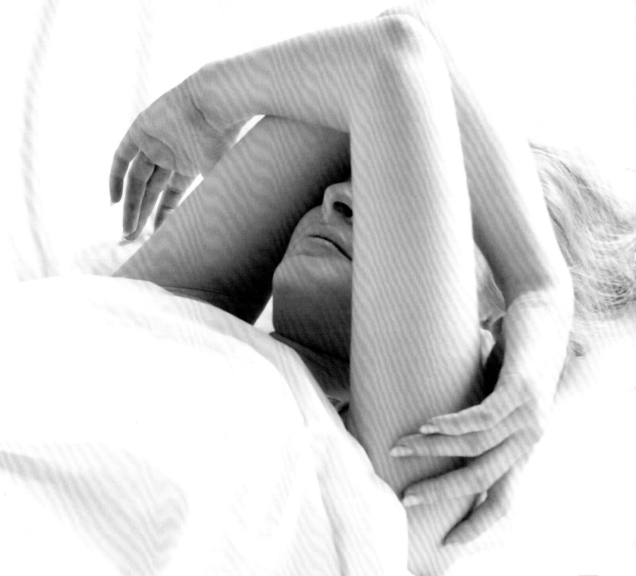

Too stressed toSLEEP?

If your racing mind is stopping you switching off at night, we've got some easy tricks for instant calm and better rest...

F eeling frazzled? You are not alone. A 2024 study showed that 77 per cent of employees felt that stress had an impact on their physical health.* Stress not only impacts how we function during the day, but also how we sleep at night. In fact, stress is often one of the top factors blamed for not getting enough shut-eye. 'Many people struggle to sleep due to stress and worries manifesting themselves during a time when they are vulnerable,' says sleep expert Dr Nerina Ramlakhan. 'Problems can seem heightened because we go into an almost childlike state when we sleep at night. There are things during the day that might not seem like a big problem, but at night they can appear a lot worse, especially during the couple of hours before bed.' Need help to get some much-needed rest during times of stress? Here's how...

Cut the caffeine earlier

'Most of us are aware that drinking a cup of coffee straight before bed is likely to keep us up at night, but many underestimate the effect that our caffeine intake throughout the day could be having on our sleep habits,' says Dr Sarah Jarvis, working with Sealy UK. 'If you're regularly struggling to nod off, try cutting caffeine out completely from lunchtime onwards to see if it has a positive effect on your sleeping habits.'

1 in 5 people in the UK aren't getting enough sleep, according to Mental Health UK.

Don't use your phone in the toilet

Always scrolling? 'When standing in a queue, we turn to our smartphones, and some people don't even go to the toilet without theirs,' says Dr Ramlakhan. 'This leaves no time for your body and mind to properly process things in our lives, so our thoughts reappear and keep the mind going, which can be a particular problem when we try to go to sleep.' If you're guilty, then schedule in smartphone downtime during the day.

Ease off the booze

'It can be tempting to have a drink or two to "unwind" before bed, especially if you're feeling stressed – but, while alcohol may help you get off to sleep, it can lead to disrupted sleep,' says Dr Jarvis. 'You're also more likely to experience rebound anxiety the next morning.'

Have a set wind-down routine

'If you have to work in the evening, stop at least an hour before you need to get to bed,' says medical nutritionist Dr Naomi Beinart. 'Write down your to-do list for the next day. Then do anything that relaxes you, such as having a bath and then reading for 20 minutes. Having a set wind-down routine helps your mind and body to let go of the day and prepare for sleep.'

Exercise at the right time

'Those who do a cardio workout at 7am sleep longer, fall into deeper sleep cycles, and spend 75 per cent more time in reparative slumber than those who work out later in the day,' says Dr Jarvis. 'Cardio workouts also elevate the body's temperature, so exercise at least three hours before bedtime in order to avoid a disrupted sleep schedule.'

And breathe...

'Forms of meditation have been proven to help relax the body and mind,' says Neil Robinson, chief sleep officer at Sealy UK. 'Slowly inhaling and exhaling will help to calm your nervous system, lower your heart rate and lead to you feeling relaxed.'

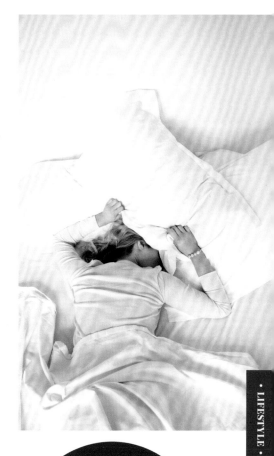

25% of UK adults admit money worries are the reason they're too stressed to sleep.**

Try this NHS-recommended breathing exercise to relax your mind and body so you can switch off...
1. Lie in bed, arms away from your sides, palms facing up.
2. Breathe deeply in through your nose, counting steadily from one to five (or as far as you can comfortably).
3. Without pausing, breathe out gently through your mouth, counting to five. Keep going for about three to five minutes.

Create a haven in the bedroom

Bedroom full of clutter? It could be adding unnecessary stress. 'Make your bed a place you enjoy spending time in, rather than dread,' says Neil. 'A comfortable healthy sleeping environment will promote deep and restful sleep.'

Herbal helpers

Need to de-stress, fast? These natural remedies can help provide relief...

✢ **Valerian root** can be bought and taken as a supplement or extract, or you can drink it as a tea to help you doze off.

✢ **Chamomile** is a popular choice as a calming tea before bed.

✢ **Lavender** can be used as an oil in a diffuser in your bedroom or as a spray on your pillow to help you relax.

Stop stressing about the time

Do you look at the clock when you wake in the night? It could be doing you more harm than you realise. 'One of the worst things people can do when they wake up during the night is to look at the clock,' says Dr Ramlakhan. This is because over-measurement of sleep, especially

Perfect pillowcase

Instead of using an oil diffuser or spraying your pillow with a herbal spray, why not try a scented pillowcase designed to help you unwind. The scented liners use aromatherapy to soothe you to sleep.

using tracking devices, is causing a new disorder called orthosomnia. 'This is where you're unhealthily preoccupied with how much sleep you are or aren't getting,' adds Dr Ramlakhan. The solution? Distract yourself. 'It's very easy to start counting down the hours until you need to be up in the morning and getting stressed as a result,' says Dr Jarvis. 'Cover up the clocks, get up and do something else in another room, such as reading a book. Once you start feeling more relaxed you can try going back to bed – sometimes a change of scene is enough to help you nod off.'

EAT YOURSELF CALMER

A healthy diet is key when your body is under pressure. 'This means eating well, staying hydrated and avoiding too much refined sugar,' says Dr Ramlakhan. Here's our daily pick...

BREAKFAST
Porridge gives you sustained energy.

MORNING SNACK
Sunflower seeds are high in magnesium to lower levels of stress hormone cortisol. 'It's known as "nature's tranquilliser" as it's associated with relaxation,' says Dr Beinart.

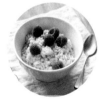

LUNCH
Cold turkey in a salad or sandwich is ideal as it contains the calming amino acid tryptophan.

AFTERNOON DRINK
Swap your 4pm cuppa for a green tea, which reduces tension-making beta

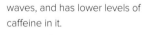

waves, and has lower levels of caffeine in it.

DINNER
Go for beef or white fish – these are high in the B vitamins needed to make feel-good serotonin. Make sure you include lots of magnesium – leafy vegetables, pumpkin seeds, buckwheat pasta, pulses and rye bread are good sources.

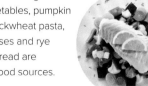

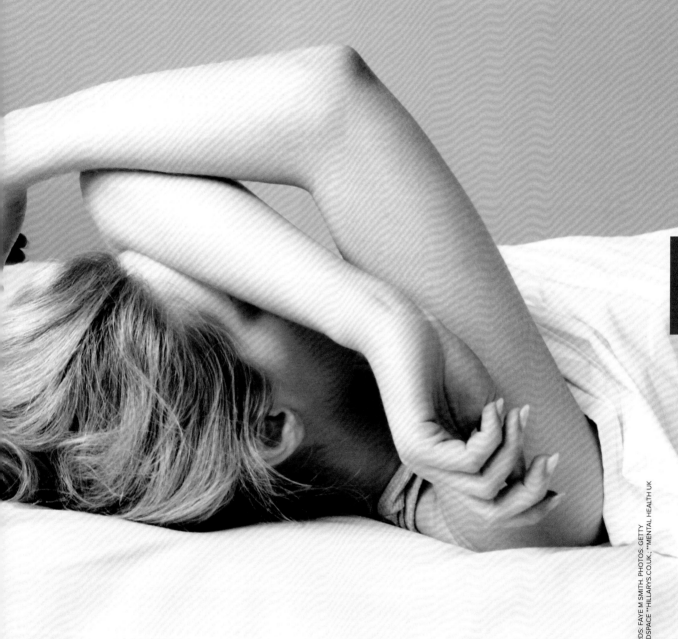

'If your stress levels are affecting your ability to cope with everyday life and you need further help, contact your GP'

· LIFESTYLE ·